Intern Mastery:

Top 10 Internal Medicine Diagnoses at the Busiest Hospitals in the Nation

Luis Daniel Lugo MD MBA

Executive Editor:

Parker Williams DO MBA

DEDICATION

This book is heartfelt dedication to my founding residents. These individuals had the option to opt for simplicity, yet they boldly chose the path of innovation, demonstrating their grit and determination. Rather than settling for what was near perfect, they made the audacious decision to create perfection themselves, embodying the true spirit of a "founder".

DISCLAIMER

Medical information in this document is not intended as a substitute for professional care. Rather, this book is meant to be an educational guide. Any recommendations provided should be integrated with the most updated guidelines and complete clinical assessment.

CONTENTS

Table of Contents

ACKNOWLEDGMENTS

In the vibrant tapestry of life, there are moments that define us, experiences that shape us, and journeys that lead us to unexpected destinations. As I pen this acknowledgement, I find myself reflecting on a journey that has been nothing short of extraordinary. From the classrooms where I taught chemistry, to the bustling hospital wards of New York where I served as a hospitalist, and later as a teaching faculty and associate program director, my path has been marked with challenges, growth, and countless learning opportunities.

The most transformative part of this journey began when I accepted the challenge of becoming the founding program director of an internal medicine residency program at Lakeland Regional Health. Uncertainty loomed, for the task of building a program from scratch was colossal, and the challenges, formidable. However, the overwhelming support and trust that I received from the senior leadership at Lakeland Regional Health made this daunting task seem achievable. Their faith in me allowed me to reshape the hospital's ED admissions workflow, transforming a hospital known for having the nation's second busiest emergency department into a beacon of academic medicine. I am grateful for their unwavering support and their commitment to creating the best internal medicine residency program in the State of Florida.

Dr. Finnigan, among her many candidates, saw potential in me and chose me to be her program director. I still vividly remember the morning I interviewed with her, shortly after the birth of my daughter. I was filled with nervous anticipation, but her trust in me emboldened my resolve. Thank you, Dr. Finnigan.

To the faculty who believed in the vision and elevated the program even before there were residents, your faith in our collective mission has been instrumental in our success. Your passion and dedication have helped shape a program that stands as a testament to the power of academic medicine, providing the hospital with some of the best quality measures in healthcare.

To the founding residents of the internal medicine program, you are the shining stars of this endeavor. You bring energy, enthusiasm, and dedication to your work every day, and I am grateful for your commitment to excellence. Your efforts have played a pivotal role in raising the bar for medical education in our region.

Lastly, but certainly not least, I would like to express my deepest gratitude to my wife. She has been a pillar of strength, her patience and understanding unwavering during the long hours and the many challenges. To her, I promise that once we have chief residents in place, things will get better. Here's to hoping that day arrives soon.

This book is a testament to the spirit of collaboration, dedication, and perseverance that has marked our journey. It serves as a beacon of hope and a testament to what can be achieved when a group of dedicated individuals come together with a shared vision. We are building something special in Lakeland, Florida, one of the fastest-growing counties in the nation. We are shaping the future of healthcare, and I am profoundly grateful to be a part of this journey.

Thank you all, for being a part of my journey, and for allowing me to be a part of yours.

Chapter I: Cardiology
Authors and Editors

Editors
Luis Daniel Lugo MD MBA
Parker Williams DO MBA

Authors
Juan Rivera Martinez MD
Aqeel Khanani DO MS
Vivek Patel MD MPH
Michael Sabina DO

Chapter I: Cardiology

Evaluation of a patient presenting with "shortness of breath and palpitations."

Mrs. J is a 67-year-old woman with a past medical history of hypertension, diabetes, and dyslipidemia who presented to the emergency department via emergency medical services for acute onset shortness of breath and occasional palpitations. The patient reported difficulty carrying groceries from her car. She reported 8-pound unintentional weight gain in the past week and was last hospitalized two years ago for shortness of breath while she was laying down at night but left against medical advice.

Pulse oximetry on presentation was 84% on room air and she was afebrile. Blood pressure was 168/98 mm Hg; pulse rate is 122/min and irregularly irregular. Cardiac examination was remarkable only for an irregular rhythm and bilateral lower extremity edema. Laboratory studies revealed an elevated B-type natriuretic peptide (BNP) and a minimally elevated high-sensitivity troponin. No acute ischemic changes were appreciated on ECG. Her systolic ejection fraction (EF) on echocardiogram was estimated to be 30% (normal >50%).

HPI Pertinent Positives

- Peripheral edema
- Orthopnea
- Shortness of breath and Dyspnea on exertion
- Weight gain
- Palpitations

Associated Comorbidities

- Coronary artery disease
- Hypertension
- Diabetes
- Dyslipidemia
- Atrial fibrillation

Heart Failure

Heart Failure (HF) is a clinical diagnosis that is characterized by symptoms such as dyspnea and fatigue, and evidence of cardiac dysfunction, which could be due to impaired ability to relax and fill with blood, eject blood, or both. Heart failure (HF) is a widespread health issue, particularly among individuals aged over 65 years in the United States. The incidence of HF has increases with age, and recent trends indicate that its prevalence is on an upward trajectory in this demographic. There are several risk factors associated with HF, including coronary heart disease, cigarette smoking, hypertension, being overweight, diabetes, and valvular heart disease. These factors significantly contribute to the increasing prevalence and incidence of heart failure.

The condition can result from various factors such as LV dysfunction, RV dysfunction, and valvular heart disease, among others. When the left ventricular ejection fraction is ≤40 percent, it is known as HF with reduced ejection fraction (HFrEF). It is worth noting that left HF is a common cause of right HF. Preventive measures should prioritize high-risk factors such as hypertension, diabetes, coronary disease, and obesity. Several major hypertension trials have indicated that treating hypertension reduces the risk of HF.

Physical Exam

- **Lower extremity swelling**: Swelling of the legs is often observed in the lower legs and ankles. Swelling caused by heart failure third-spacing is pitting in nature, compared to non-pitting edema seen in peripheral vascular disease. For individuals confined to the bed, swelling may also appear in the sacral area and upper thighs. Documentation of peripheral edema should include grade (up to 4+), pitting nature, and superior most location of pitting. A Deep Venous Thrombosis (DVT) should be suspected in the case of unilateral pitting edema.
- **Weight gain**: Nonspecific finding caused by fluid retention. It is often acute, over days to weeks.
- **Rales (crackles) on pulmonary exam**: Fluid overload contributes to the development of pulmonary edema; fluid accumulates in the lung interstitium and surrounding alveoli, resulting in the presence of rales on auscultation. The absence of crackling sounds (rales) doesn't necessarily mean there is no pulmonary vascular congestion. Rales are generally best heard at the base of each lung & should be auscultated directly over skin.
- **Elevated jugular venous pressure**: Fluid overload associated with right-sided heart failure leads to increased pressure in the venous system causing notable distension of the jugular veins in the neck.
- **Cough**: Classically with pink, frothy, or rusty colored sputum. Caused by fluid accumulation in the lungs, especially when the patient is supine.

- **Hepatojugular reflux**: Fluid congestion in the venous system can lead to engorgement of the liver. As a result, pressure on the liver via palpation forces fluid back into visible neck veins.
- **Abdominal distention**: Nonspecific finding due to fluid retention. Commonly seen in right heart failure due to left ventricular dysfunction.
- **S3 Heart Sound**: In heart failure, the ventricles dilate, stiffen and become less compliant. As a result, the early filling of these ventricles requires more pressure, which leads to increased turbulence. This produces an extra heart sound, S3, during diastole. The presence of this S3 indicates reduced ventricular compliance and elevated filling pressure.

Laboratory Data

- **Plasma BNP values above 400 pg/mL**: Ventricular stretch from chronic volume overload triggers the release of BNP from cardiomyocytes as a reflex and compensatory mechanism to promote vasodilation and diuresis. Notably, this value may be falsely normal in obese patients and varied in those with CKD. For patients in sacubitril/valsartan, a pro-BNP is more reliable (sacubitril increases levels of BNP). Trending of BNP and pro-BNP are tempting but offer little clinical utility.
- **Cardiac Troponin or high-sensitivity Troponin**: Myocardial oxygen demand-supply mismatch can cause myonecrosis, which then releases troponin into the circulation. Though elevated levels suggest ischemia, troponins can be elevated in heart failure without myocardial ischemia. And this can be potentially helpful regarding risk stratification. Subendocardial ischemia, wall stress, and endothelial dysfunction all play a role in troponin elevation.
- **Liver Function Tests**: Hepatic vein congestion secondary to right heart failure can be reflected by elevations in these liver function tests.
- **Serum Sodium**: HF with reduced ejection fraction can lead to low renal perfusion. This activates RAAS and vasopressin release, causing sodium and water retention, with has the effect of diluting serum sodium. Studies associate hyponatremia with increased rates of rehospitalization, prolonged hospital courses, and even greater rates of mortality.
- **Serum Creatinine**: Acute elevations in creatinine levels are indicative of low renal perfusion and are generally resolved with correction of the underlying problem of heart failure.

Imaging Findings

- **Chest X-ray**
  - **Cardiomegaly**: Enlarged cardiac silhouette, with a cardiac to thoracic width ratio > 50% is commonly observed. The presence of a "Boot-shaped" heart on PA view of CXR is associated with RV enlargement.
  - **Pulmonary Edema**: Fluid from leaky capillaries floods the interstitial and alveolar spaces in the lungs due to the elevated pulmonary venous pressures secondary to left heart failure.
- **Electrocardiogram**
  - Acute ST segment changes or Q waves suggest ischemia as the possible cause of HF.
  - Persistent ST elevations suggest LV aneurysm as the cause of HF.
  - Ventricular hypertrophy suggests diastolic HF.
  - Abnormal p waves suggest dilated left atrium as the possible cause of HF.
  - Conduction delays, such as LBBB.
- **Transthoracic Echocardiography**
  - Preserved LV ejection fraction: Impaired LV relaxation (diastolic function) causing decreased end diastolic volume thus increased filling pressure which leads to backflow into the left atrium and pulmonary veins.
  - Reduced LV ejection fraction: Impaired cardiac contractility (systolic function) of the LV leads to reduced ejection of blood into the aorta thus, backflow into the left atrium and pulmonary veins.
  - Right ventricle dilation: LV failure causes pulmonary hypertension and resulting increased RV afterload. This chronically leads to RV dilation and dysfunction.
  - Left Heart Valvopathy
    - Aortic stenosis leading to poor systolic function and chronically causing LV hypertrophy (diastolic dysfunction)
    - Mitral stenosis will create decreased EDV and backing up flow into LA and pulmonary circulation.
    - Aortic/Mitral regurgitation
  - Right Heart valvopathy
    - Pulmonary/tricuspid stenosis/regurgitation

Diagnostic Workup

The diagnostic approach of acute decompensated heart failure remains pivotal from the constellation of clinical symptoms and signs. Hence, initial assessment should include a brief, focused history and a physical examination to evaluate signs and symptoms of HF (**as described above**) as well as potential contributing factors and comorbidities. These signs can be further supported by appropriate investigations, such as ECG, chest radiograph, biomarkers (B-type natriuretic peptide [BNP] or N-terminal proBNP [NT-proBNP]), and transthoracic echocardiography.

The clinician should start with a thorough history and physical exam, looking for key symptoms like orthopnea, paroxysmal nocturnal dyspnea, and edema, as well as exam findings like elevated jugular venous pressure, pulmonary rales, S3 heart sound, and peripheral edema. These clinical findings suggest heart failure, and a chest X-ray looking for pulmonary edema and cardiomegaly, an ECG to evaluate for LVH and ischemia, and lab tests like BNP which are elevated in heart failure. If clinical suspicion remains high, the clinician should process to a transthoracic echocardiogram to evaluate ventricular function and filling pressures, which would help confirm the diagnosis of systolic and diastolic heart failure; additionally, this would provide estimates of left ventricular ejection fraction to help further differentiate the type of heart failure: reduced EF vs preserved EF. Additional testing like stress test, cardiac catheterization, or even an endomyocardial biopsy may be considered if the etiology remains uncertain.

- **Differential Diagnoses to Consider**
  - Pulmonary embolism
  - Pulmonary effusion
  - Cardiac tamponade
  - Pneumonia
  - Cardiac arrythmia
  - Asthma/COPD

Treatment

- Discontinue medications that are known to exacerbate congestive heart failure, such as non-dihydropyridine calcium channel blockers. PDE-5 inhibitors and pioglitazones are also known to exacerbate CHF but should be discontinued on admission.
- Restrict fluid intake, especially in those with severe exacerbation.
- Diet low in salt
- Treatment via GDMT (Goal Directed Medical Therapy)
  - Combination therapy preferred over maximizing single agent.
- Oxygen therapy as needed.
  - Used in patients in which acute or chronic hypoxia is present. If the patient is saturating 90% or more, we hold the oxygen.

- Loop Diuretics
  - Before starting diuresis, we take in consideration the creatinine and previous treatment with loop diuretics. A cutoff creatinine of 2, is generally used.
  - In patients that has never received loop diuretics in the past, initial doses consist of IV furosemide 20 mg to 40 mg, IV Torsemide 10mg to 20 mg, or IV Bumetanide 1 mg. We can start administration every 12 hours, but the dose can be increased to every 8 hours, as needed. Volume status must be considered.
  - In patients receiving loop diuretics as part of their medication regimen, generally, the initial dose will be at least 2x dose (eg, patients receiving daily oral furosemide 40 mg at home, the initial dose will then be IV furosemide 40 to 80 mg). If the patient is not responding as expected, diuretic resistance may be considered, and the dose may be further increased. Nephrology consultation should also be considered.
- Vasodilators
  - Nitroglycerin is generally used when loop diuretics alone are not sufficient to reduce preload, the amount of fluid returning to the heart.
  - Nitroprusside can be used in patients with severe hypertension. Remember that this medication is associated with cyanide toxicity. Strict monitoring is required.
- Inotropes
  - For severe exacerbations, dopamine, dobutamine, or milrinone may be considered.

Intern Mastery

- **Clinical Documentation**
  - Accurate documentation of the type of heart failure is important and provides clarity to all providers caring for the patient.
  - Decompensated Systolic Congestive Heart Failure vs Diastolic vs Combined.
    - Acute vs Chronic vs Acute on Chronic.
  - Do not diagnose HF on a single EF. Consider clinical history and document accordingly e.g.
    - Heart Failure with EF improved from reduced range to preserved range.
    - Heart Failure with EF improved from reduced range to mildly reduced range.
  - Consider additional documentation of Ischemic vs

  - Nonischemic CM if present and NYHA class.
    - Heart Failure with Reduced Ejection Fraction HFrEF (<40%).
    - HFimpEF (EF >40% after being below 40%).
    - HFmrEF (EF 40-49%).
    - HFpEF (EF >50%).

- **Monitoring**
  - Daily I's & O's may inform you if the patient is having effective diuresis. The goal is to have a patient on a net negative total fluid balance every day.
  - Daily weights can also cue us in to assessing patient's total fluid status. The goal is for the patient to lose weight progressively with effective diuresis.
  - Studies examining the impact of therapy guided by BNP or NT-proBNP on clinical outcomes in patients with chronic heart failure have yielded inconsistent results. The majority of the evidence hints that there may be little to no significant improvement when drug treatment for heart failure is adjusted based on natriuretic peptide levels.

- **Discharge Planning**
  - Education on weight monitoring, diet, and medication compliance.
  - Patient education should focus on dietary modifications, such as restricting sodium and fluid intake: recommend following a low-sodium diet (less than 2 grams per day) and limiting total daily fluid intake to 1.5 to 2 liters.
  - Discuss daily weight monitoring and signs of fluid overload to look out for, such as increasing edema or shortness of breath.
  - Instruct patients on when to notify their physician for symptoms refractory to diuretics. Regular outpatients follow up to determine adequate maintenance diuretic dose, rescue dose, and potential need for K supplementation.
  - Arrange a cardiology or primary care physician follow-up within two weeks for discharge for medication titration, weight checks, symptom monitoring, and for device diagnostics review if patient has an ICD.
  - Strongly reinforce additional lifestyle modifications such as tobacco cessation and regular exercise routines to improve overall physical conditioning.

- **Guideline: ACC/AHA and the recommended treatment for chronic HFrEF**.

- Decrease mortality and hospitalizations.
    - RAS/neprilysin inhibitors or RAS inhibitors:
        - Preferred: sacubitril-valsartan (ARNI)
        - Alternatives: ACE/ARBs inhibitors
        - Wait at least 36 hours to start ARNI after discontinuing ACE-I/ARB.
    - B blockers: Benefits NYHA I-IV by reducing mortality.
        - Preferred: Metoprolol Succinate, Carvedilol, and Bisoprolol have proven mortality benefit (metoprolol tartrate does not).
    - Aldosterone antagonist
        - Preferred: Spironolactone, Eplerenone
        - Initiate if GFR >30
            - Eplerenone has less instances of gynecomastia as side effect and can be started if GFR >20
        - There's new data on Finerenone and how it "Reduces Risk of Incident Heart Failure in Patients With Chronic Kidney Disease and Type 2 Diabetes." Finerenone is a novel selective, nonsteroidal mineralocorticoid receptor antagonist.
    - SGLT2 inhibitors: decrease death from HF hospitalization.
        - Preferred: Dapagliflozin, Empagliflozin
        - Alternative: Canagliflozin
        - GFR of 30 or more required for dapagliflozin, GFR of 20 or more required for empagliflozin.
- Do not decrease mortality but can reduce hospitalizations and improve symptoms:
    - Hydralazine plus Nitrates:
        - For patients with NYHA class III-IV, and who cannot tolerate ACE/ARB inhibitors. May reduce mortality in African Americans.
    - Ivabradine
        - Consider in patients with persistent symptoms, on maximum B-blocker therapy, NYHA class II-III, EF of 35% or less, and a heart rate of 70 of greater.
    - Digoxin: Decrease hospitalizations.
        - Indicated in patients with Heart failure + afib refractory to BB and ACEi.
        - Monitor potassium and digoxin levels regularly.
    - Vericiguat: Vasodilator
        - Can be used on top of primary therapy for patients with Heart failure.

- - No significant reduction in all-cause mortality or hospitalizations.
  - Avoid nondihydropyridine calcium channel blockers (diltiazem or verapamil) as they may be harmful to HFrEF.
- Cardiac resynchronization therapy
  - AKA biventricular pacing
  - Indicated in patients with EF of 35 or less with NYHA class II or IV symptoms despite maximal GDMT + LBBB with QRS of 150ms or greater.
- Implantable cardiac defibrillator
  - Indicated in patients with EF of 35 or less with NYHA class II or III symptoms despite maximal GDMT.
  - In patients with NYHA class IV, can be indicated if patient is heart transplant candidate or with LVAD.
  - Avoid proceeding with the implantation of an ICD until after three months of guideline-directed medical therapy has been administered, or 40 days post-myocardial infarction. This waiting period is important to evaluate the potential recovery of left ventricular ejection fraction (LVEF).
- Iron supplements
  - Iron deficiency anemia independently associated with severity of heart failure.
  - Guidelines recommend IV iron therapy in patients with IDA as opposed to oral due to possibility of poor gut absorption.
- Anticoagulation
  - No evidence of benefit in isolated HF.
- Novel med therapy
  - Omecamtiv Mecarbil: Myotope that acts on sarcomere by increasing number of myosin heads, thus more pulling on actin filaments creating greater force during systole.
  - Per ACC, no reduction in mortality, but there was a decrease in hospitalizations.

Challenge Questions

1. Which medications must be avoided in patients with decompensated HFrEF?
   a. **B-blockers**

    b. Calcium channel blockers
    c. Nitrates

2. Which of the following does not increase BNP?
    a. Kidney failure
    b. Older age
    c. Female sex
    d. Obesity

3. Which of the following best describes the New York Heart Association (NYHA) functional classification system for heart failure?
    a. A system based on left ventricular ejection fraction (LVEF)
    b. A system based on age and gender
    c. A system based on symptom severity and functional limitations

Atrial Fibrillation

This is the most commonly treated arrhythmia in the United States. Individuals with atrial fibrillation (AF) face elevated risks of mortality, heart failure, hospitalization, and thromboembolic events. Although AF usually advances from paroxysmal to persistent stages, individuals may experience both types over time. Valvular AF pertains to patients with moderate to severe mitral stenosis, and these individuals are at an increased risk of stroke. AF should not be confused with multifocal atrial tachycardia (MAT), an arrythmia commonly seen in patients with chronic obstructive pulmonary disease (COPD). Notably, the United States Preventive Services Task Force (USPSTF) abstains from recommending screening for AF.

Physical Exam

- **Irregularly irregular pulse**: The chaotic electrical activity of the fibrillating atria sends erratic conduction to the AV node. As a result, there are irregular R-R intervals that may be appreciated with evaluating patients' pulses.
- **Tachycardia**: The electric impulse produced in the SA node reaches the ventricles faster when the atria is not contracting properly. This is called a fib with rapid ventricular response.
- **Presence of heart murmurs**: If atrial fibrillation is caused by heart failure, an S3 or S4 can often be present, and noted on auscultation.
- **Goiter and exophthalmos**: If present in a patient with atrial

fibrillation, suggests hyperthyroidism as the most likely cause.

Laboratory Data

- **Complete blood count (CBC)**: A CBC should be considered; signs of infection or anemia may precipitate atrial fibrillation.
- **Basic Metabolic Panel (BMP)**: Electrolyte imbalances can be a contributing factor to atrial fibrillation as well.
- **TSH and T4**: Low TSH and a-fib suggests hyperthyroidism as the most likely cause.
- **Urine drug screen**: Cocaine and amphetamines are a common cause of atrial fibrillation, and tachycardias in general.
- **Ethanol**: Elevated levels of ethanol in the blood can be indicative of binge drinking, a known cause of atrial fibrillation. This is known as Holiday Syndrome.

Imaging Findings

- **Chest X-ray**
  - Vascular congestion: Chronic atrial fibrillation causes enlargement of the left atrium, which eventually increases backflow pressure to the pulmonary vasculature.
  - Enlarged cardiac silhouette.
- **Electrocardiogram**
  - Absent P waves: The P wave represents atrial depolarization. P waves are absent because depolarization is impaired, causing lack of true atrial contraction through the cardiac cycle.
  - Irregular R-R waves: The distance between two adjacent R waves is not consistent.
- **Doppler Echocardiography**
  - Enlarged left atrium: chronic atrial fibrillation causes electrical and structural remodeling of the atria. Over time, this leads to LA enlargement that can be appreciated on echocardiograms.
  - Reduced left ventricular function: rapid heart over time can exceed the myocardium's capacity, cause tachycardia-induced cardiomyopathy, which then leads to reduced left ventricular function as downstream effects.
- **Sleep Study**
  - Identifying and treating underlying sleep disorders can significantly improve the management of atrial fibrillation.

Diagnostic Workup

The key test is an electrocardiogram looking for absence of P waves, irregular R-R intervals, and fibrillatory waves, which confirm this arrhythmia. The clinician should also elicit relevant history like presence of palpitations, varying pulse intensity, and consider risk factors like hypertension and age. An echocardiogram helps determine if the atrial fibrillation has caused cardiomyopathy, while also identifying the presence of comorbid valvular disease. Extended or ambulatory ECG monitoring documents and records these episodes when outpatient, while exercise testing can provoke atrial fibrillation episodes for closer monitoring.

As described above, laboratory analysis useful in the diagnosis of atrial fibrillation include TSH and urine drug screening tests. Hyperthyroidism, thyrotoxicosis, alcohol intoxication, cocaine use, and amphetamines use are well known to be associated with atrial fibrillation. A sleep study may also be considered.

- **Differential Diagnoses to Consider**
  - Atrial fibrillation
  - Atrial Flutter (classic sawtooth P waves, usually 2:1 conduction, rate ~300 bpm)
  - Multifocal Atrial Tachycardia (>3 P wave morphologies, irregular rate, classically seen in COPD)
  - Sinus Tachycardia
  - Atrial Tachycardia

Treatment

The treatment of atrial fibrillation is dependent on onset and the patient's hemodynamic stability. Hemodynamic instability due to unstable atrial fibrillation often presents with refractory hypotension, cardiogenic shock, or myocardial ischemia. In these patients, emergent synchronized electrical cardioversion is indicated to normalize these patients' rhythms.
  - If new onset and less than 48 hours, can cardiovert without AC.
  - If RVR and need pressors, consider phenylephrine due to reflex bradycardia.

In hemodynamically stable patients, treatment is dependent on the onset of atrial fibrillation. Patients with onset greater than 48 hours should be treated with rate control initially, using agents such as beta-blockers (metoprolol, atenolol, propranolol) or calcium channel blockers (diltiazem, verapamil). Consideration of rhythm control agents should be deferred until thrombi can be ruled out via transesophageal echocardiogram (TEE) or following 3 weeks of anticoagulation. Second- and third-line rate control options include digoxin and amiodarone, respectively.

Patients with new onset atrial fibrillation with an onset less than 48 hours, can be treated **with either rate control** (e.g. metoprolol or diltiazem) **or rhythm control** using antiarrhythmics such as amiodarone, sotalol, flecainide, and others.

Given the high risk described, oral anticoagulation with Coumadin is always considered for Valvular Atrial Fibrillation.

Intern Mastery

- **Clinical Documentation**
  - Accurate documentation of the type of atrial fibrillation is important and provides clarity to all providers caring for the patient.
  - New Onset Atrial Fibrillation with Rapid Ventricular Response vs Atrial Fibrillation.
  - Paroxysmal AF: AF of 7 days or less.
  - Persistent AF: AF of >7 days.
  - Long-standing persistent: Persistent AF that lasts >1 year.
  - Permanent AF: Persistent that has not been able to be restored to sinus rhythm.
  - Silent or Asymptomatic AF: Incidental diagnosis without symptoms.

- **Monitoring**
  - External event monitors or implantable loop recorders can be used to detect asymptomatic AF episodes and monitor response to treatment. 24-48 hour continuous ECG monitoring is useful for quantifying AF burden and response to therapy.
  - Symptom monitoring – Patient's should journal AF symptoms of palpitations, fatigue, or shortness of breath to help the patient correlate symptoms of AF with episodes.

- **Discharge Planning**
  - Educate the patient on classic symptoms of atrial fibrillation such as palpitations, lightheadedness, or shortness of breath and when to seek urgent medical care.
  - Discuss the importance of adherence to anticoagulation therapy like warfarin or direct oral anticoagulants (DOAC) to

> reduce risk of stroke. Warfarin should be used for anticoagulation in patients with valvular AF (moderate or severe mitral stenosis or mechanical valve prosthesis), not a DOAC.
>
> - Encourage moderation of alcohol, caffeine, and stress, which are known to trigger atrial fibrillation episodes. Advise other lifestyle modifications such as staying well-hydrated.
> - Coordinate follow-ups as needed with electrophysiology to evaluate for ablation therapy if needed. Consider referral to establish care with pulmonology and/or sleep medicine to control other exacerbating factors like sleep apnea.
> - Schedule follow-up with cardiology in 1-2 weeks to assess symptoms, titrate medications, and review ambulatory ECG monitoring data.

- **Guideline: Professional medical societies and the recommended treatment for Atrial Fibrillation**.
    - Rate control: for most patients, achieving a resting heart rate of less than 80 bpm is recommended (AHA/ACC/HRS, 2019).
    - Preferred: Metoprolol Succinate > Tartrate
        - Alternative: Verapamil and Diltiazem. Used in severe COPD (where B blockers are contraindicated).
            - Diltiazem Can increase digoxin levels.
            - Verapamil can worsen HF in patients with LV dysfunction.
        - Special situations: Consider Digoxin in HF or low blood pressure, or Amiodarone.
    - Rhythm control: for symptomatic patients refractory to rate control medications use antiarrhythmics (AHA/ACC/HRS, 2019).
        - Class IA: Procainamide. Cautions: Increase in QT interval, can cause low blood pressure.
        - Class IC: Flecainide, Propafenone. Contraindicated in patients with structural or ischemic heart disease.
        - Class III: Amiodarone, Dronedarone, Ibutilide, Sotalol. Cautions: increase in QT interval.
    - Cardioversion: In patients with persistent AF this is the long-term management strategy. TTE done prior to rule out embolism in atrial appendage or in one of the heart chambers. Cardioversion can precipitate a thromboembolic event if clot is present.
    - Ablation: If younger than 80 years old with persistent AF with unsuccessful cardioversion or AF recurrence (1-3 months after CV)
    - Anticoagulation: A-fib provoked by valvular disease, require oral anticoagulation. Use the $CHA_2DS_2\text{-}VAS_c$ for patients with Non

valvular A fib. Anticoagulate if ≥1 and no contraindications.
- o Preferred: Rivaroxaban, Apixaban, Edoxaban (Factor Xa inhibitors).
- o If GFR <15 or on dialysis can use warfarin or apixaban.
    - If serum creatinine ≥1.5 or ESRD on dialysis: renally dose apixaban to 2.5 mg BID if patient is ≥80 or weighs <60kg.
- o Alternatives: Dabigatran (thrombin inhibitor), Warfarin (require continuous laboratory monitoring to maintain INR 2-3), Watchman device.
    - Weigh risk of major bleeding with oral anticoagulation via HAS-BLED scoring system. If risk of bleeding higher than risk of stroke use clinical judgement and shared decision making.

Challenge Questions

1. What are two conditions in which warfarin is recommended over NOAC (Non-vitamin K antagonist oral anticoagulants)?
    a. Mild mitral stenosis, CKD
    b. **Moderate/severe mitral stenosis or mechanical heart valve**
    c. Mitral regurgitation and rheumatic heart disease
    d. Atrial stenosis and mitral regurgitation

2. What is one of the most common causes of atrial fibrillation, and most of the time goes unnoticed?
    a. Hyperthyroidism
    b. Alcohol induced
    c. Advanced age
    d. **Obstructive sleep apnea**

3. Which organs can be affected by Amiodarone? (Select all that apply)
    a. Heart
    b. **Lungs**
    c. **Liver**
    d. Thyroid

Hospital Course

In the ED, Mrs. J was given three doses of IV metoprolol q5minutes with little response. Subsequently, she was started on IV Cardizem and Heparin for AF with rapid ventricular response and suspected acute decompensated heart failure, unknown EF. The patient was admitted to the med-tele floor and started on IV diuresis with furosemide. On POCUS exam, LVEF was estimated to be low. Over the next 48 hours, her heart rate was tightly controlled in the 80s. Repeat EKG showed resolution of rapid ventricular response. On hospital day 3, Mrs. J was successfully transitioned from IV Cardizem to oral Metoprolol. Her CHADS2VASC score was calculated at 5, she was transitioned to Apixaban for stroke prevention. By hospital day 5, the patient was euvolemic on oral diuretics and remained in normal sinus rhythm. Patient improved towards baseline and was discharged home on Metoprolol, Furosemide, Atorvastatin, Entresto and Apixaban with cardiology follow-up. An SGLT-2 was recommended.

Chapter II: Pulmonology
Authors and Editors

Editors
Luis Daniel Lugo MD MBA
Parker Williams DO MBA

Authors
Aqeel Khanani DO MS
Adrian Feliciano MD
Christopher Fitts MD
Samuel Belgique MD

Chapter II: Pulmonology

Evaluation of a patient presenting with "progressive difficulty ambulating"

Mr. F is a 65-year-old male with a past medical history of poorly-controlled hypertension and type 2 diabetes mellitus who presented to the ED with a one-week history of progressive shortness of breath and increasing difficulty performing daily activities of living. He reported gradual worsening over the last few weeks, and he now finds it difficult to perform even mild physical activities without becoming severely breathless. He is a former smoker with a 40 pack-year history and quit 4 years ago. He reported chills, wheezing, fatigue, productive cough with green sputum, and pleuritic chest pain on deep inspiration. His family also noticed recent loss of appetite. He denied any recent travel or sick contacts.

His vitals revealed a temperature of 101.5°F (38.6°C), blood pressure of 140/90 mmHg, heart rate 110 bpm, respiratory rate 24 bpm, and oxygen saturation 90% on 2 L oxygen by nasal cannula. Examination revealed decreased breath sounds, wheezing and crackles on auscultation over the bilateral lower lung field. CBC showed leukocytosis (WBC: 15,500/mm³), hemoglobin: 13.2 g/dL, and platelet count: 290,000/mm. Chest X-ray showed a dense consolidation on bilateral lower lobes.

HPI Pertinent Positives

- Cold and flu-like symptoms
  - Sore throat / rhinorrhea / fatigue, malaise / chills
- Fever [oral temp >100.4 F (38 C)]
- Cough (productive vs dry) and Shortness of breath
- Sputum production (clear vs blood-tinged vs green vs rust-colored)
- Smoking pack year status

Associated Comorbidities

- Diabetes
- Hypertension

Chronic Obstructive Pulmonary Disease (COPD) Exacerbation

COPD is an obstructive lung disease primarily associated with a greater than 10 pack-year smoking history. Chronic Obstructive Pulmonary Disease (COPD) is a significant global health issue, ranking as the third leading cause of death worldwide in 2019. Exacerbations are often triggered by factors such as infection, pollutants, GERD, chronic bronchitis, or climatic changes and result in a sudden and sustained deterioration of respiratory symptoms, lung function, and quality of life. Symptoms of an exacerbation include difficulty breathing, coughing, wheezing, tightness in the chest, and producing more mucus. Notably, exacerbation rates and overall mortality are typically higher during winter. Additionally, early fatalities among hospitalized patients with severe COPD exacerbation are often due to concurrent conditions like pulmonary embolus, pneumonia, or congestive heart failure. These patients may also face an elevated risk of myocardial infarction and stroke following an exacerbation.

Although COPD is clinically diagnosed through pulmonary function testing, patients who present to the hospital with suspected COPD exacerbation based on smoking history and clinical picture are often treated empirically. An exacerbation can be very dangerous and may require hospitalization. Hypoxemia is treated with escalating oxygen and ventilation assistance, hypercapnia is treated with BiPAP, and intravenous steroids and breathing treatments form the backbone of treatment. Future exacerbations can be prevented by following the individualized treatment plan, quitting smoking, getting vaccinated, and staying away from irritants.

- Classically COPD is a grouped diagnosis consisting of asthma, chronic bronchitis, bronchiectasis, and emphysema. We when diagnose, or expect someone to have an exacerbation of COPD, these are the underlying disease processes we need to be thinking of. The treatment is very similar amongst these diseases, however, there are specific treatment options that might be considered if we know exactly what disease is causing the patient's symptoms.
- Radiological studies will be of great assistance to us when determining the diagnosis. We will discuss below the specific findings of asthma, chronic bronchitis, bronchiectasis, and emphysema via different imaging techniques. Most of this will be kept at a basic level of interpretation, however, your institutional radiologists are always a phone call away for further discussion of in-depth concerns of your patients.
- Imaging of an Asthmatic
    - The best first imaging technique is a chest x-ray. This is for several reasons; they are cheap, very low radiation exposure, quick, can be done at bedside if needed, give us enough imaging findings to make quick differentials and treatment plans. CT chest will always give more anatomical definition, ability to differentiate between disease

processes; however, its more radiation, patient must be moved to the scanner, can take longer for a full reading from radiologist and more expensive.

o   Radiological findings of an uncomplicated asthmatic are typically due to diffuse airway narrowing. This leads to hyperinflation of the lungs causing large lung volumes, flattening or even an inversion of the diaphragm, marked attenuation of the peripheral vascular markings. Additionally, you can see bronchial inflammation and thickening causing a peribronchial cuffing which can sometimes appear as "tram-tracking." These findings are seen on chest x-ray as well as CT chest.

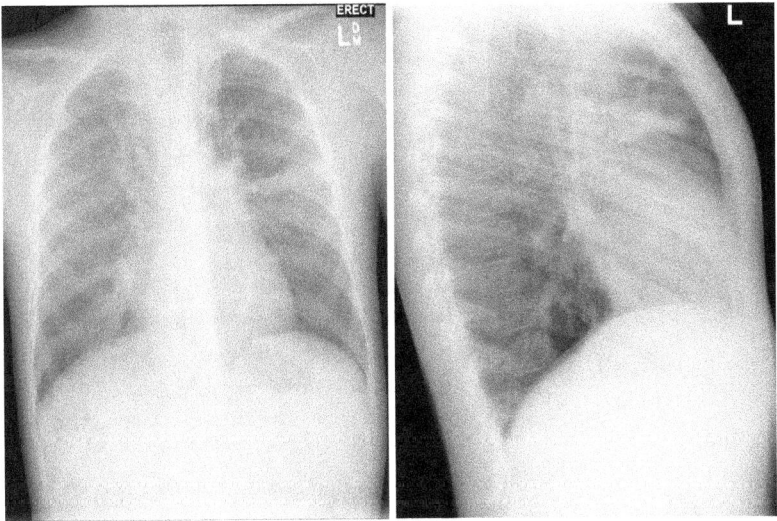

- Chronic Bronchitis is typically defined as a clinical diagnosis rather than an imaging diagnosis. You will look for excess mucous production, expectoration of the mucous on most days for at least 3 consecutive months with at least 2 consecutive years. Imaging these patients can be completely normal. In fact, approximately 50% of patients who have a history of chronic bronchitis have completely normal chest x-rays.

    o   If there are radiological changes, you can see similar changes as those asthmatic patients. Commonly, peribronchial cuffing or "tram-tracking" can be seen when there is bronchial inflammation or thickening. In other patients, they can have what is referred to as "dirty chest" which shows up as accentuated peripheral lung markings.

This finding isn't directly correlated to a specific pathophysiological finding; however, it does appear there is loose correlation with thickened airway walls, smoking related small airway disease. CT chest can show clear bronchial wall thickening and/or presence of mucous plugging.

- Emphysema
    - o An abnormal enlargement of the airspaces which are beyond the terminal bronchioles and typically permanent. You will get destruction of the alveoli which is typically without an obvious fibrotic process.
    - o Two different classifications: centrilobular and panlobular. Centrilobular is typically the most common and can be diagnosed as destruction of the central portion of the pulmonary lobule. Most often, centrilobular affects the upper lobes. Panlobar is a less common form of emphysema and causes a uniform distention of the airspaces throughout the entirety of the pulmonary lobule. This form of emphysema typically will affect the lower lobes of the lung.
    - o Radiological studies and findings
        - ▪ Frontal and lateral chest x-rays are the most common starting point.
        - ▪ Findings: diffuse hyperlucency (panlobular emphysema) caused by the destruction of the capillary bed as well as the alveolar septi. A flattening and possible depression of the diaphragm associated with an increased retrosternal airspace caused by loss of the elastic recoil of the lung parenchyma resulting in hyperinflation. Bulla which are caused due to the alveolar thin walls and destruction of adjacent alveoli. Increased peripheral vascular markings can be seen as well. This is more commonly seen in the centrilobular form. This is caused by the small airways being damaged with a subsequent increase in the pulmonary vascularity.

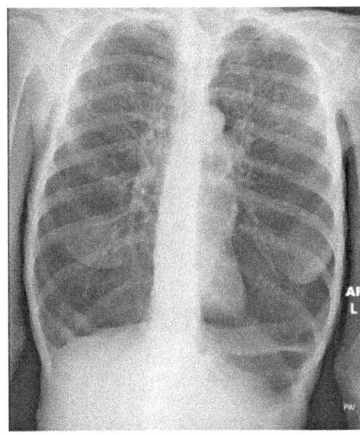 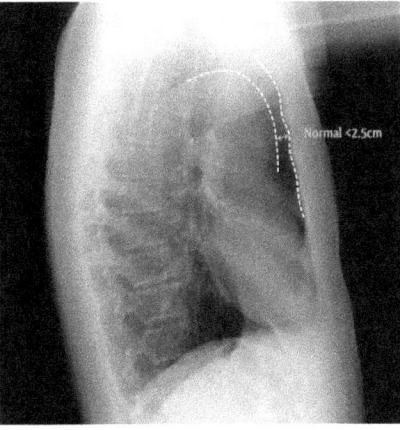

Physical Exam

- **Increased respiratory rate**: A rate greater than 20 breaths/minute indicates increased work of breathing, which is often observed within this group of patients.
- **Wheezing on auscultation of lungs**: High-pitched whistling sound during breathing suggests ongoing bronchoconstriction.
- **Accessory respiratory muscle use**: Contraction of neck, chest, and abdominal muscles to assist in breathing is often seen as these patients display increased work of breathing.
- **Tripod positioning**: A sign of increased work of breathing as patients sit hunched forward with arms on knees to optimize chest expansion.
- **Prolonged expiratory phase**: Chronic airway obstruction in these patients leads to longer periods of expiration.
- **Distended jugular veins**: It may be observed in advanced disease states as a sign of right heart strain from COPD-related pulmonary hypertension.
- **Diminished breath sounds**: Decreased air entry from bronchospasms or secretion-related obstructions.

Laboratory Data

- **Leukocytosis**: The white blood cell (WBC) count of a patient with an acute exacerbation of COPD may vary depending on the cause and severity of the exacerbation. If the exacerbation is caused by a bacterial infection, the WBC count may be elevated, indicating an inflammatory response. Bacteria like S. pneumoniae and H. influenzae are known to stimulate intense neutrophilic inflammation. The bronchial and alveolar irritation induces cytokine release and chemotaxis of white blood cells.

If the exacerbation is caused by a viral infection, the WBC count may be normal or slightly decreased, reflecting viral suppression of bone marrow function.

- **Eosinophilia**: If the exacerbation is caused by environmental factors, such as air pollution or allergens, the WBC count may not change significantly. A rise in eosinophils can point to an allergic or inflammatory response to environmental irritant that may have precipitated the exacerbation. Inhaled allergens, dust, or air pollution can activate eosinophilic inflammation in the airways.
- **Elevated Hematocrit**: Due to chronic hypoxemia, the kidneys respond by increasing erythropoietin to chronically produce more red blood cells. Hematocrit further rises during episodes of acute exacerbations as more RBCs are released from vasoconstriction in hypoxic lung tissues.
- **Arterial Blood Gas (ABG) abnormalities**:
  - Respiratory acidosis: elevated $PaCO_2$ (hypercapnia) due to impaired gas exchanged caused by increased airway resistance and reduced alveolar ventilation.
  - Hypoxemia: decreased PaO_2 due to ventilation-perfusion (V/Q) mismatch and impaired diffusion caused by airway obstruction and inflammation.
- **Elevated C-Reactive Protein (CRP)**: CRP is an acute phase reactant and levels rise in response to inflammation, reflecting the systemic inflammatory component of COPD exacerbations.

Imaging Findings

- **Chest X-ray (CXR):**
  - Hyperinflation: increased lung volumes due to air trapping and reduced expiratory flow is a hallmark of COPD. This results from chronic airway inflammation, bronchoconstriction, and chronic/progressive loss of lung elasticity.
  - Flattened diaphragms: diaphragmatic flattening occurs due to hyperinflation and increased work of breathing. This compromises the diaphragm's contractile efficiency and contributes to respiratory muscle fatigue
  - Bullae: big pockets of air that develop in the lung tissue when alveoli are damaged. They look like areas of low density with fewer blood vessels, and they usually affect the upper lobes of the lungs.
  - Small, vertical heart: The heart is narrow and elongated due to the compression by the hyperinflated lungs and can be seen as a narrowed cardiac silhouette.

Diagnostic Workup

When diagnosing a COPD exacerbation, it is essential to begin with a comprehensive assessment that includes a detailed medical history and thorough physical examination. The history must include patient's smoking history, previous COPD diagnoses, current medications, and recent respiratory infections or exacerbations. In the physical examination, attention should be given to the patient's general appearance and the degree of respiratory distress. Lung auscultation is crucial to identify characteristic findings like wheezing, crackles, or decreased breath sounds. Additionally, observing the use of accessory muscles and checking for signs of cyanosis or cor pulmonale, such as jugular venous distention and lower extremity edema, helps in gauging the severity of the exacerbation.

Routine laboratory tests should be conducted, including a complete blood count (CBC) to assess for an elevated white blood cell count, which could suggest infection, and to monitor hematocrit levels for polycythemia. A basic metabolic panel (BMP) should be obtained to check for electrolyte imbalances, particularly potassium levels if bronchodilators are part of the treatment plan. An arterial blood gas (ABG) analysis is crucial for assessing oxygenation (PaO_2) and ventilation ($PaCO_2$), which provide valuable information for determining the severity of respiratory failure and directing treatment decisions.

Key diagnostic tests include a chest X-ray (CXR) to evaluate lung hyperinflation, rule out other potential causes of acute respiratory symptoms such as pneumonia, and identify complications like pneumothorax. Sputum cultures can identify bacterial infections triggering the exacerbation. Cardiac workup is important to rule out heart failure, which can mimic COPD flares. NT-proBNP, EKG, and echocardiography help distinguish cardiac versus pulmonary causes of dyspnea. These components of the diagnostic workup ensure a comprehensive assessment of the patient's condition, guiding appropriate treatment strategies and interventions for COPD exacerbation management. In summary, a multi-modal approach is required, including thorough physical examination, routine labs, chest imaging, arterial blood gases, sputum cultures, and cardiac testing when appropriate.

- **Differential Diagnoses to Consider**
  - Pneumonia
  - Heart Failure Exacerbation
  - Pulmonary Embolism

- Asthma Exacerbation
- Interstitial Lung Disease

Treatment

Initial Assessment and Stabilization

- Evaluate vital signs, respiratory rate, oxygen saturation, degree of dyspnea, and for signs of respiratory distress (accessory muscle use, tripoding, speaking in broken sentences)
- In patients with Chronic Obstructive Pulmonary Disease, provide supplemental oxygen to maintain saturation above 88%. Start with a low-flow oxygen device like nasal cannula and titrate flow rate to reach target saturation levels.

Medication Management

- Initiate treatment with short-acting bronchodilators, such as short-acting beta-agonists (SABA) like albuterol or short-acting anticholinergics (SAMA) like ipratropium. These can be administered via a nebulizer or metered-dose inhaler with a spacer.
- Administer systemic corticosteroids, typically prednisone, to reduce airway inflammation. In the outpatient setting, the usual dose is 40-60 mg orally daily for 5-10 days. In the inpatient setting, we may use intravenous methylprednisolone.
- Consider antibiotics if there is evidence of increased sputum purulence, a change in sputum color, or signs of infection. The choice of antibiotics should be based on local resistance patterns.

Intern Mastery

- **Clinical Documentation**
  - Accurate documentation COPD is important and provides clarity to all providers caring for the patient.
  - COPD vs. Acute Exacerbation of COPD
  - vs. Acute Exacerbation of COPD with Pneumonia
  - vs. Acute Exacerbation of COPD with Acute Hypoxic Respiratory Failure

- **Monitoring**
  - When a patient presents with an acute exacerbation of COPD, as the physician, you will need to ensure close monitoring and prompt treatment. Assess the patient's respiratory status frequently, checking their oxygen saturation, respiratory rate, use of accessory muscles, and mental status. Titrate oxygen to maintain saturations

between 88-92%. If the patient is in respiratory distress, check arterial blood gases to guide oxygen therapy and evaluate for respiratory failure. Listen for wheezes, rhonchi, or crackles with frequent lung auscultation. Use chest imaging to identify complications such as pneumonia. Monitor the patient's mental status for signs of hypercapnic encephalopathy, and check ABGs for indications of hypercapnia.

- If the patient has a productive cough, observe sputum character and send a sample for culture if you suspect an infection.
- Evaluate the patient's response to bronchodilators and steroids through lung re-examination and pulmonary function testing. Periodically monitor blood glucose levels as hyperglycemia can occur with steroid treatment. Consider pulmonary medicine consultation should the patient not improve under these measures.

- **Discharge Planning**
  - Confirm patient has remained clinically stable with improved respiratory status: no worsening hypoxemia, tachypnea, or respiratory distress.
  - Ensure education: Patient demonstrates correct use of inhalers, nebulizers, oxygen if needed.
  - Ensure patient has appropriate discharge medications: bronchodilators, steroids, and antibiotics if prescribed. Review written discharge instructions on COPD care, medication use, and when to seek emergency medical attention.
  - Prescribe and arrange home oxygen if oxygen saturations remain low with ambulation.
  - Schedule follow up appointment with primary care physician within 1-2 weeks of discharge.
  - Encourage smoking cessation if patient smokes.

- **Guideline: 2023 Global Initiative for Chronic Obstructive Lung Disease (GOLD) report provides clinical recommendations on the management of acute COPD exacerbations.**
  1. GOLD's updated 2023 definition of a COPD exacerbation is an event characterized by increased dyspnea, cough and/or sputum that worsens within 14 days, may be accompanied by tachypnoea and/or tachycardia, and is often associated with an increased inflammatory state due to insults to the airways such as infection, allergens, or pollutants.
  2. Inhaled short-acting beta-2-agonists administered are the first-line bronchodilators used for the acute management of COPD exacerbations.

3. The use of systemic glucocorticoids via prednisone 40 mg is recommended for management of COPD exacerbations to restore lung function and improve oxygenation. Whether PO or IV, it is recommended to administer a five-day course of treatment, keeping in mind that longer courses may worsen mortality rates.
4. Indications for the administration of antibiotics amidst a COPD exacerbation include cases in which patients present with increased sputum purulence and/or volume. In these instances, the antibiotic therapy should be targeted and last for 5 to 7 days.

Challenge Questions

1. In what scenario is non-invasive positive pressure ventilation (NIPPV) typically indicated in patients with COPD exacerbations?
   a. Hypoxemic respiratory failure
   b. Hypercapnic respiratory failure
   c. Mild dyspnea
   d. Stable COPD

2. What key components of post-hospitalization care are important for patients with COPD exacerbations to reduce the risk of readmission and improve their quality of life?
   a. Encouraging smoking cessation
   b. Prescribing long-term antibiotics
   c. Discontinuing all medications
   d. Providing home oxygen therapy

3. What is recommended to be checked on all patients with COPD?
   a. Procalcitonin
   b. Bicarbonate
   c. Alpha-1 Antitrypsin level
   d. Hematocrit level

Bacterial Pneumonia

In the United States, 25 out of every 10,000 adults are diagnosed with pneumonia every year. Pneumonia is more common among aging populations, is a major cause of death, and often requires intensive care unit level care. The death rate for these patients can be up to 23%. Anaerobic infections are uncommon causes of Community-acquired pneumonia, but should be considered in patients not responding to standard pharmacotherapy. Streptococcus pneumoniae is among the most common pathogens causing pneumonia. Mycoplasma pneumoniae is among the most common pathogen causing atypical pneumonia.

Physical Exam

- **Increased respiratory rate**: Tachypnea, body attempts to compensate for impaired lung.
- **Decreased breath sounds**: The affected lung field may be heard upon auscultation.
- **Crackles or rales**: Fine crackling sounds, can be heard on lung auscultation usually during inspiration due to the presence of fluid or mucus in the airways.
- **Dullness on percussion**: It indicates consolidation of localized area.
- **Pleural friction rub**: It may be associated with a pleural effusion.
- **Enhanced bronchophony**

Laboratory Data

- **Complete blood count (CBC)**: A CBC should be considered; signs of infection with increased white blood cell count, bandemia, or leukopenia may be present.
- **Sputum culture and Gram Stain / Respiratory Pathogen Panel**
- **Inflammatory markers**: Markers like C-reactive protein (**CRP**) or **Procalcitonin** may assist in the diagnostic workup.

Imaging Findings

- **Chest X-Ray**
  - **Lobar Pneumonia (A)**
    - **Opacity** of one or more pulmonary lobes
    - Presence of air bronchograms
      - translucent bronchi inside opaque areas of alveolar consolidation
  - **Bronchopneumonia (B)**
    - Poorly defined **patchy infiltrates** scattered throughout the lungs
    - Presence of air bronchograms
  - **Atypical or interstitial pneumonia (C)**
    - Diffuse **reticular opacity**
    - Absent (or minimal) consolidation

A, B and C below, respectively.

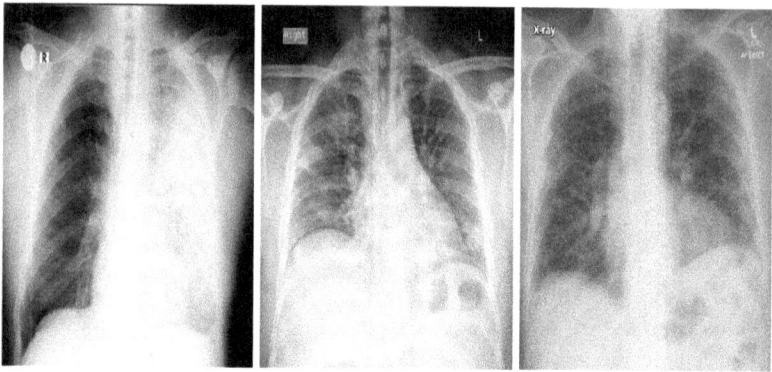

- **Chest CT (usually without contrast)**
  - Ordered to further evaluate the extent of lung involvement or assess for complications like lung abscesses.
  - Indications: Inconclusive chest x-ray / Recurrent pneumonia / Poor response to antibiotics

Diagnostic Workup

The diagnostic workup for bacterial pneumonia involves clinical assessment, imaging, and lab tests. It starts with a thorough patient history to understand symptoms and risk factors. A focused physical exam, including lung assessment, is performed. A chest X-ray (CXR) is often used to confirm the diagnosis, but if it's inconclusive and clinical suspicion remains high, a chest CT or empirical treatment may be considered. Lab tests include a complete blood count (CBC) for signs of infection, sputum cultures for identifying the bacteria, and markers like procalcitonin or C-reactive protein (CRP) for inflammation levels. In severe cases, an arterial blood gas (ABG) helps assess oxygenation. A useful tool for guiding decisions regarding hospital admission is the Pneumonia Risk Score (CURB-65), which considers factors such as confusion, blood urea levels, respiratory rate, blood pressure, and age to assess the severity of pneumonia and aid in making informed decisions about patient care.

- **Differential Diagnoses to Consider**
  - COPD or Asthma Exacerbation
  - Heart Failure exacerbation
  - Drug-induced pneumonitis
  - Pulmonary interstitial fibrosis
  - Pulmonary Embolus or Infarction
  - Septic Emboli in patients with bacterial endocarditis

Treatment

Outpatient Setting

Five days of antibiotic therapy is usually prescribed and any patient being treated in a primary care setting should be re-examined after 48–72 hours to evaluate the efficacy of the prescribe antibiotic.

Inpatient Setting

The course may vary depending on the patient's response, but it may usually range between 7-10 days of a broader spectrum antibiotic. You may consider longer courses in patients not responding to treatment, concerns for MRSA or P. aeruginosa infection, concurrent meningitis, or unusual pathogens.

Additional considerations: Anaerobic coverage is not routinely recommended for suspected aspiration pneumonia (unless lung abscess or empyema is suspected). Despite growing evidence, corticosteroids are not routinely recommended as adjunct therapy.

Intern Mastery

- **Clinical Documentation**
    - Accurate documentation of the type of pneumonia is important and provides clarity to all providers caring for the patient.
    - Pneumonia secondary to (specify GRAM positive/negative – confirmed pathogen)
    - Typical vs Atypical / Bacteria vs Viral Pneumonia
    - Sepsis (if present) secondary to bacterial (specific) pneumonia

- **Monitoring**
    - Vitals signs should be closely monitored to assess for decompensation or worsening into sepsis. Review patient's inflammatory markers and assess for any presence of end organ damage.
    - Procalcitonin $\geq$ 0.25 mcg/L correlate with an increased probability of a bacterial infection. Low levels may help in the decision to discontinue antibiotics. It's used as a tool to guide antibiotic treatment but not to decide if treatment should be started.

- **Discharge Planning**
    - Unless there's a specific indication, as the patient improves, antibiotics should be transitioned from antibiotic to oral.
        - For patients with uncomplicated CAP who

demonstrate rapid defervescence and clinical improvement over the first 3 days, a 5-day course of therapy is adequate for cure.

- There's data advocating for shorter antibiotic courses. Every patient needs antibiotics to be tailored to their needs. Educate the patient on the importance of completing the antibiotic treatment to avoid readmission.
- Patients should follow up with their primary care physician within 1-2 weeks to assess for improvement and/or resolution. Strict return to hospital precautions (recurring fevers, worsening of symptoms) should be given on discharge.

- **ID Clinical Guidelines**
  - Patients should be counseled to quit smoking, abstain from alcohol intoxication, and maintain dental hygiene.
  - The Pneumonia Severity Index (PSI) and Infectious Disease Society of America/American Thoracic Society (IDSA/ATS) scoring systems help predict site of care.
  - There are two types of vaccines that may protect patients from pneumonia: PPSV 23 and PCV 13. These vaccines work against different types of bacteria that cause pneumonia. People who are 65 years or older or who have a higher risk of getting pneumonia should get both vaccines. Here are the guidelines for when and how to get the vaccines:
    - For individuals aged 19 to 64 without immune compromise, start with PPSV 23, then at age 65, get PCV 13 one year after the first PPSV 23 dose, followed by another PPSV 23 dose at least five years later.
    - If you're 19 to 64 with immune compromise or asplenia, begin with PCV 13, followed by PPSV 23 eight weeks later, and another PPSV 23 dose five years after the first.
    - For those 65 and older without prior vaccines, initiate with PCV 13, followed by PPSV 23. If immune-competent, wait one year between vaccines, or eight weeks if immune-compromised or asplenic.
    - Consider an annual influenza vaccine, especially if at higher risk for flu complications, as the flu can lead to or worsen pneumonia.

Hospital Course

With this past medical history, recent fevers, worsening respiratory function, and increased sputum purulence, Mr. F was promptly admitted to the hospital with a diagnosis of COPD exacerbation and sepsis secondary to bacterial pneumonia. He was started on empiric antibiotic therapy with ceftriaxone and azithromycin. In addition, he received nebulized bronchodilators, IV methylprednisolone, and supplemental oxygen therapy to address his COPD exacerbation. Mr. F's condition gradually improved. He remained in the hospital for a total of 7 days, during which he completed a course of antibiotics and systemic corticosteroids. After careful monitoring and rehabilitation, he was discharged home with a follow-up plan for pulmonary rehabilitation and close outpatient monitoring to manage his COPD and continue his recovery from pneumonia.

Challenge Questions

1. In which of the following cases are glucocorticoids recommended in patients with community-acquired pneumonia?
   a. Patients with severe COPD
   b. Patients with history of adrenal insufficiency
   c. Patients with Stage IV HFrEF
   d. Patients with refractory septic shock

2. Patient presenting with bacterial pneumonia caused by MRSA but is allergic to Vancomycin. PGY-1 resident starts Daptomycin treatment. Is this the correct drug of choice in this scenario?

   a. Yes, Daptomycin covers MRSA pneumonia.
   b. No, Daptomycin does not work on lung due to inhibition by surfactant.
   c. No, give Vancomycin even though there are allergies to medication.
   d. No, will consider starting antibiotic treatment with Piperacillin-Tazobactam

3. When patient has ongoing fever due to suspected bacterial pneumonia with no medical improvement despite optimal/correct medical treatment of antibiotic. Which of the following is the most appropriate step in management?
   A) Obtain sputum cultures, repeat chest X-ray, and consider broadening antibiotic regimen.
   B) Bronchoscopy with biopsy
   C) Thoracentesis with drainage, possible chest tube placement
   D) Same antibiotic regimen but for a longer duration

Chapter III: Infectious Diseases
Authors and Editors

Editors
Luis Daniel Lugo MD MBA
Parker Williams DO MBA

Authors
Emma Weiland MD
Graciela Luna MD
Bryce Green DO
Zein Barakat DO MS

Chapter III: Infectious Diseases

Evaluation of a nursing home patient with "fever and altered mental status."

Mr. K is 85-year-old male with a medical history of poorly controlled type 2 diabetes complicated by peripheral neuropathy, hypertension, peripheral vascular disease, and benign prostatic hyperplasia s/p transurethral prostate resection (TURP) who presented to the emergency room with chief complaints of subjective fever and acute onset confusion determined by the staff at his skilled nursing home (SNF). Upon questioning, he reported occasional chills and flank pain. The patient had a recent TURP and was sent to his SNF with an indwelling urinary catheter at that time. New onset "confusion" and urinary symptoms developed over the next 24 hours after the nursing staff noticed blood in urinary catheter bag. Of note, patient also reported worsening swelling of his left leg.

Vitals revealed tachycardia, tachypnea but normotension. On exam, there were erythematous streaks extending proximally from a localized area on the lateral aspect of his left leg. The area was erythematous, swollen and tender. Bright red blood was also appreciated in the Foley bag. Urinalysis was remarkable for blood and nitrites and significant white blood cells.

HPI Pertinent Positives

- Altered mental Status / Confusion
- Hematuria
- Flank pain
- Recent procedure
- Dysuria
- Presence of Indwelling Foley catheter
- Rash localized to the lateral left leg

Associated Comorbidities

- Poorly controlled type 2 diabetes mellitus complicated by peripheral neuropathy and peripheral vascular disease
  - At risk for various complications, including diabetic foot infections. Neuropathy can lead to a lack of sensation in the affected areas, which may delay recognition of infections.
- Benign prostatic hyperplasia s/p TURP

Urinary Tract Infections (UTI)

Community acquired urinary tract infections are one of the most common infections requiring treatment with antibiotics. UTIs account for approximately 40% of all nosocomial infections; most of these are in association with the use of long-term urinary catheter usage. A majority of acute uncomplicated UTIs occur in women aged 18-24 years. UTIs are considerably less common in men under the age of 50, and, if suspected, should prompt further workup for the cause. Escherichia coli is the causative pathogen for approximately 80% of all UTIs. Other pathogens such as staphylococcus aureus, enterococci, gram negative bacilli such as proteus, Klebsiella, Serratia, and Pseudomonas species are most typically seen in complicated urinary tract infections.

A complicated UTI may be defined as an infection that goes beyond the bladder (ie, UTI with fever or other systemic symptoms, pyelonephritis, and/or UTI with sepsis or bacteremia).

Physical Exam

- **Suprapubic tenderness**
- **Costovertebral angle tenderness**: This may be indicative of pyelonephritis, perinephric abscess, or renal calculi.

Lab Findings

- **Complete blood count (CBC)**: A CBC should be considered; signs of infection with increased white blood cell count, bandemia, or leukopenia may be present.
- **Basic Metabolic Panel (BMP)**: There may be evidence of kidney injury/elevated creatinine.
- **Beta hCG**: This must be done in all women of childbearing age who have not previously undergone a hysterectomy or tubal ligation. This is imperative when considering imaging and treatment modalities.
- **Urinalysis with reflex culture**: Ideally, via clean catch/straight catheter.
- **Blood cultures:** This is usually considered in elderly or hospitalized patients with sepsis and critically ill patients.

Imaging Findings

Most imaging studies are reserved for patients who are acutely ill, those with signs of sepsis/shock, or if signs of urinary tract obstruction/abscess formation are present.

- **Kidney and bladder ultrasound**
  - The preferred initial study
- **Computed tomography with and without contrast**
  - For patients with ultrasound findings of anatomic abnormality or pyelonephritis
  - Can identify prostatitis, renal calculi, obstruction, abscesses, or other gas forming infections.

Diagnostic Workup

The first step is to assess the overall stability of the patient. In the unstable patient, intravenous fluids and empiric antibiotic treatment should be initiated promptly following appropriate cultures are collected. Cultures can guide treatment and improve outcomes. Urinalysis should be obtained, preferably using a straight catheter or clean catch (not from existing catheter), prior to initiation of antibiotics. Antibiotics should not be delayed.

In the stable patient, the focus is directed first to the history, as this is vital to determining disease diagnosis and classification for appropriate treatment. Urinary tract infections can be classified as uncomplicated or complicated and can involve variable portions of the urinary tract. Ultimately, proper treatment is determined by the likelihood of infection, the potential source of infection, and the likelihood that the patient is infected with a resistant organism, which are often acquired in a healthcare setting. A good history can elucidate the potential organism causing the UTI.

UTIs are classified as acute non-complicated and acute complicated UTI.

- **Acute non-complicated cystitis**
  - Noncomplicated cystitis is an infection that is confined to the bladder. This is most commonly caused by colonization of the urethra by fecal floral pathogens. Typically, patients will present with symptoms such as urinary frequency, urinary urgency, dysuria, hematuria and suprapubic pain. Any symptoms of vaginal discharge or pruritis should prompt a pelvic examination to rule out vaginosis, STIs or PID.
- **Acute complicated UTI (fever/pyelonephritis/etc.)**
  - A complicated UTI is an infection that travels beyond the

bladder to the ureter(s) and kidney(s). There are several risk factors which include: male sex, pregnancy, immunocompromised, renal transplant recipients, indwelling urinary catheter, or poorly controlled diabetes mellitus. The typical symptoms include fever/chills, rigors, fatigue, headache, nausea, vomiting, flank pain, costovertebral angle tenderness, and pelvic pain. The signs of a noncomplicated cystitis may or may not be present.

If the patient clinically deteriorates and remains clinically symptomatic after 48-72 hours or if a urinary tract obstruction is suspected, imaging studies and blood cultures are warranted.

- CT abdomen and pelvis with and without contrast
- Blood cultures

Urinalysis interpretation

When interpreting a urinalysis to rule out urinary tract infection, it is important to first assess how the sample was collected and whether or not it may be contaminated by external bacterial flora. Ideally, samples should be collected via clean catch or straight catheter to avoid contamination. One of the best indicators of contamination is the presence of epithelial cells.

- If the method of collection is adequate and epithelial cells are minimal, the presence of bacteria, leukocyte esterase, nitrites, and white blood cells are interpreted together to assess the likelihood of urinary tract infection.
- If none of the 4 are present, a urinary tract infection is highly unlikely, antibiotics are generally not given and another cause for the symptoms should be investigated.
- If a urinary tract infection is suspected based on the aforementioned findings, a reflex culture should be triggered if ordered. Generally, cultures can take days to weeks to grow out and sensitivities can take longer. Below are the common macroscopic and microscopic descriptor see with urinalysis.

Macroscopic Urinalysis

- **Appearance**: Clear, cloudy or turbid are common descriptors, and all can potentially be considered normal. Cloudy urine can be caused by sperm, epithelial cells, elevated protein, RBCs, WBCs and bacteria. Changes in appearance can also be due to dehydration, urinary tract infections, nephrolithiasis, diabetes and sexually transmitted diseases.
- **Color**: Commonly ranges from colorless or pale yellow to a deep

amber color. However, certain disease processes, bacteria, food and dietary supplements can affect the color.

- o Brown coloration can be seen in the presence of bile pigments, melanin and methemoglobin.
- o Red coloration could be indicative of hematuria, hemoglobinuria, myoglobinuria or porphyria.
- o Green coloration could indicate pseudomonas.

- **Specific Gravity:** Normal values range from 1.007 - 1.030. This shows the concentration of the particles within the urine. Abnormalities can be seen in many disease processes from Addison Disease, diabetes, heart failure, dehydration, renal artery stenosis, SIADH. UTIs will usually cause an elevation.

- **Glucose:** If seen in the urine, is considered a non-specific finding. This can be seen in patients with hyperglycemia, diabetes, pregnancy, certain medications such as SGLT2 inhibitors.

- **Bilirubin:** Is usually detectable in very small amounts within the urine. Any elevation seen within the urine are generally indicative of liver or bile duct pathology.

- **Ketones:** Ketones are usually negative; however, these can also be a normal finding for a subset of patients. When seen in the urine, it can be indicative of the body breaking down fats and fatty acids to use as a source of fuel for the body. Ketones are commonly elevated in diabetic ketoacidosis, with fasting, in patients following a very low carbohydrate diet, or with the use of SGLT2 inhibitors.

- **Blood:** This is usually negative. It should be noted that this is reported separately from RBCs, which are reported under the microscopic examination. While positive blood in the urine can mean RBCs, it can also be indicative of dehydration, exercise, hemoglobinuria, myoglobinuria, or menstrual bleeding. If positive, it is imperative to evaluate how the urine was collected and to consider other potential causes.

- **pH:** The normal range is typically 4.5 – 8.0. An elevated urine pH (>8.0) may indicate kidney disease or UTI, while a low urine pH (<4.5) may indicate DKA or diarrhea.

- **Protein:** Less than 30 mg per day is normal. The most common protein found in urine is albumin. Elevated protein is commonly seen in heart failure, kidney injury and dehydration.

- **Bilirubin:** Bilirubin is usually undetectable, or is only seen in small amounts. If detected, it is usually conjugated (direct) bilirubin as this is the water-soluble form. Elevation should prompt further evaluation for possible liver dysfunction or biliary obstruction.

- **Urobilinogen:** Small amounts can be normally seen in the urine. Any elevation can be indicative of hepatocellular disease or hemolysis.

- **Nitrites**: A normal urine with be negative for nitrites; however, a negative level does not fully exclude the possibility of a urinary tract infection. Bacteria you can expect to see in a nitrate positive urine are the gram negatives such as E.coli, Klebsiella, Enterobacter or Proteus.
- **Leukocyte Esterase**: Normally negative for most patients. Leukocyte esterase is an enzyme that is present on most WBCs, thus if positive, is an indicator of an increased number of WBCs. Positive leukocyte esterase and nitrites together is highly predictive for UTI.

Microscopic Urinalysis

- **RBCs**: Less than 3/hpf is considered normal. The presence of RBCs is always abnormal and may require further evaluation. Contamination from hemorrhoids, or vaginal bleeding can occur. Alternatively, this can be indicative of kidney/ureter/bladder cancer, urinary tract infections and nephrolithiasis.
- **WBCs**: Less than 5/hpf is considered normal. A positive test or elevation in WBCs usually indicates infection, inflammation, or bacterial colonization within the urinary tract.
- **Epithelial cells**: Some epithelial cells within a urinalysis is considered normal; however, if there are more than 15 squamous epithelial cells, contamination of sample should be suspected. Elevation can otherwise be indicative of cancer, inflammation, or infection.
- **Bacteria**: Presence of bacteria commonly indicates an acute infection, but this is not always the case, nor is treatment always necessary. While urine is sterile, once catheterization or urologic instrumentation has occurred colonization can occur. Colonization will be discussed separately.
- **Casts**: Originate from the distal convoluted tubule or collecting duct of the kidney. Specific casts can be indicative of various disease processes.
  - Hyaline casts are mucoproteins and can be indicate pyelonephritis or CKD.
  - Red Blood Cell casts can be normal in individuals that play contact sports, but can also be indicative of glomerulonephritis.
  - White Blood Cell casts, if seen, should point you toward glomerulonephritis, interstitial nephritis, pyelonephritis or other renal inflammatory diseases.
  - Epithelial casts are cells from the renal tubule. These can be

seen in acute tubular necrosis, nephritic syndrome, eclampsia, interstitial nephritis, heavy metal ingestion, and allograft rejection.
- Waxy or Granular casts are indicative of CKD.
- Fatty casts, which are lipid-laden cells of the renal tubule can point to CKD, hypothyroidism, and nephritic syndrome.

Macroscopic	Normal	Abnormal
Blood	Absent	+ or -
Nitrite	Absent	+ or -
Leukocyte Esterase	Absent	+
Microscopic	**Normal**	**Abnormal**
RBC	<3/hpf	+ or -
WBC	<5/hpf	>5/hpf
Bacteria	Absent (usually)	+
Epithelial cells	<15	Absent or few

Urine culture

- Urine culture should be ordered as a reflex with urinalysis in patients with acute complicated UTI, urinary symptoms and male sex, poorly controlled diabetes, history of multidrug resistant infection, inpatient stay in hospital or nursing home, recent antibiotic use, recurrent UTI, and presence of indwelling urinary catheter. A positive culture would indicate 100,000 colony forming units (CFUs)/ml, and will further determine the causative organism and antimicrobial susceptibility. Susceptibility can detect which antibiotic works best by inhibiting bacterial growth. If non-susceptibility to one agent in 3 or more antimicrobial categories, MDRO infection is diagnosed.
- **Non-pathogenic bacteria**
  - Lactobacilli
  - Corynebacterial species,
  - Gardnerella
  - Alpha-hemolytic streptococci
  - Aerobes
- **Most common cause of UTIs in women**
  - Escherichia coli
- **Common pathogenic bacteria**
  - Enterobacter
  - Streptococci particularly agalactiae

- Enterococci
- Staphylococci particularly saprophyticus
- **Hospital-acquired species**
  - Enterobacter
  - Klebsiella
  - Morganella
  - Citrobacter
  - Serratia
  - Pseudomonas
- Staphylococcus aureus found in isolation is particularly indicative of recent instrumentation or as an external source such as endocarditis.

- **Differential Diagnoses to Consider**
  - Vaginitis
  - Urethritis
  - Pelvic inflammatory disease
  - Acute bacterial prostatitis
  - Nephrolithiasis
  - Interstitial cystitis or Painful bladder syndrome

Treatment

- **Acute simple cystitis/Uncomplicated UTI**
  - In the outpatient setting, if a patient presents with signs and symptoms suggesting non-complicated acute cystitis and no risk factors such as past history of MDRO infection, hospital stay, use of antibiotics in the past 3 months, therapy may start empirically without a urine culture.
  - First line agents:
    - Nitrofurantoin monohydrate/microcrystals 100mg PO BID for 5 days

or

- TMP/SMX DS 160/800mg PO BID for 3 days
  - Second line agents:
    - Amoxicillin-Clavulanate 500mg PO BID for 5-7 days

or

- Cefpodoxime 250mg PO BID for 5-7 days
  - Third line agents:
    - Ciprofloxacin 250mg BID or 500mg QD for 3 days

or

- Levofloxacin 250mg PO QD for 3 days

In addition to antibiotics, patients with severe dysuria can be given a urinary analgesic such as phenazopyridine up to 3 times a day for symptomatic relief. However, this should not be used chronically as it could mask symptoms of future UTIs.

- **Acute complicated UTI: Inpatient Treatment**
    - IV fluids to be started, as well as empiric antibiotic coverage and adjustment after urinary culture results. Treatment is given for 10-14 days.
o   Empiric gram negative coverage
    - Ceftriaxone 1g IV q24h

or

    - Piperacillin-tazobactam 3.375g IV q6h

Evaluating the hospital's antibiogram for antibiotic resistance and understanding institutional protocols is crucial. This knowledge can aid in formulating the best effective treatment, preserving patient safety, and combating the growing challenge of antibiotic resistance.

Intern Mastery

- **Clinical Documentation**
    - Accurate documentation of the type of urinary tract infection is important and provides clarity to all providers caring for the patient.
    - Severe acute urinary tract infection secondary to Escherichia coli complicated by pyelonephritis and hematuria.
    - Indicate complicated vs. uncomplicated
    - Complicated UTI infections carry increased risk of treatment failure:
        - Immunocompromised patients
        - Any UTI in males
        - UTI associated with fever, SIRS, sepsis, shock, stones, obstruction, or catheters
        - Presence of anatomic abnormalities
        - Atypical organisms
        - Recurrent infections despite adequate treatment, multi-drug resistant organisms
        - Infections in pregnancy
        - Infections after urinary tract any instrumentation or surgical intervention

- Infections after renal transplant or spinal cord injuries
- Kidney involvement: dialysis patients, impaired renal function, anuria
- Indicate the stage, severity, acuity and episode
- Indicate symptomatology
  - Symptomatic (e.g. dysuria) vs asymptomatic bacteriuria
- Mild, moderate or severe
- Acute vs chronic vs acute on chronic
- Initial episode vs recurrent vs treatment resistant
- Indicate if present on admission (POA)
- Importance is to avoid being dinged for causing a CAUTI.
- Indicate any associated conditions
- Indicate the suspected organism
  - "due to", "with" or "secondary to"
- Is the UTI causing SIRS, sepsis or shock
- Any history of previous bacteria treated and if susceptible vs resistant in past
- Indicate associated complications
  - Cystitis, pyelonephritis or hydronephrosis if present
  - Laterality if relevant (ex. Bilateral hydronephrosis)
  - Document any strictures or calculus obstructions

- **Monitoring**
  - Pregnant patients and acute cystitis
    - Obtain urine culture to confirm eradication of the bacteriuria
    - Repeat urinalysis and cultures at specific time intervals throughout pregnancy
  - Patients with acute pyelonephritis or prostatitis
    - Repeat urinalysis and culture to confirm eradication
    - Treat any recurrences
  - Consultation
    - Complications of cystitis and pyelonephritis
    - Patients with indwelling catheters/catheter use
    - Urology
      - Obstructing stone with concurrent UTI
      - Outlet obstruction
      - Recurrent UTIs of unknown cause
    - Interventional Radiology
      - Pyelonephritis secondary to obstructing stone in the renal pelvis or ureter
      - These patients may require nephrostomy tube

placement prior to stone removal

- **Discharge Planning**
  - Education on risk factors for UTI: sexual activity, pregnancy, age, poor hygiene, anatomic abnormalities
  - Prevention
    - Urinating after sexual activity
    - Increasing fluid intake, adequate hydration
    - Wiping techniques and hygiene strategies to prevent fecal flora from colonizing the bladder via the urethra
    - Benefit of showers over baths for genital hygiene
    - Vaginal estrogen used for postmenopausal females
    - Preventative antibiotics for those who repeatedly develop bladder infections
  - Medications
    - Oral antibiotics for completion of course as described in treatment section
    - Over the counter cranberry juice or cranberry tablets for prevention
  - Outpatient follow up may not needed in uncomplicated patients for whom the symptoms resolved with adequate treatment. It is required for high-risk patients, pregnant patients, or patients with complications of pyelonephritis, prostatitis, abscess formation or if upcoming urologic procedure.

- **Guideline: IDSA 2019 Management of Asymptomatic Bacteriuria Recommendations:**
    - Screen pregnant women for and treat ASB
    - 4-7 course of antimicrobial treatment for pregnant women
    - Do not screen or treat ASB in functionally impaired residents of long-term care facilities
    - Do not screen diabetic patients for ASB
    - Do not screen renal transplant patients > 1 month after surgery
    - In patients with high risk neutropenia, we make no recommendation for or against screening
    - Screen patients who will undergo endoscopic urologic procedure with mucosal trauma

Challenge Questions

1. What is the first best step in treatment of a patient suspected of

having a catheter associated urinary tract infection (CAUTI)?
   a. Start empiric antibiotics on the patient
   b. Remove the indwelling catheter
   c. Repeat a urinalysis with culture
   d. Wait for antibiogram before starting antibiotics

2. When is treatment for asymptomatic bacteriuria indicated?
   a. Pregnant women
   b. Patients undergoing urologic procedures
   c. Both a and b
   d. Neither a nor b

3. A 31 year old female presents with fever, nausea, and flank pain. BP 98/62. On labs, her urinalysis is positive and culture grows E. coli. What is the best treatment plan?
   a. Oral ampicillin for 10 days
   b. Oral trimethoprim-sulfamethoxazole twice daily for 5 days
   c. Oral nitrofurantoin four times a day for 5 days
   d. Initially IV and then oral ciprofloxacin upon discharge for 14 days total

Cellulitis

Cellulitis is a common skin and soft tissue infection (SSTI) characterized by acute inflammation of the dermal and subcutaneous tissues. It can be classified into purulent and non-purulent (or simple) cellulitis, with the latter being more common. Purulent cellulitis involves pus formation and often implicates Staphylococcus aureus. Diabetic foot infections often involve polymicrobial infections and may extend to bones (osteomyelitis). Management requires both antibiotic therapy and wound care, with amputation as a last resort.

Physical Exam

- **Skin Erythema**: Cellulitis typically presents with an area of redness on the skin, which may be warm to the touch.
- **Swelling**: The affected area often appears swollen or edematous. The skin may also feel warmer than the surrounding tissue due to inflammation.
- **Pain**: Patients may experience pain or tenderness in the affected area.
- **Fever**: Some patients with cellulitis may develop a fever as a systemic response to infection.
- **Skin Texture**: The skin over the affected area can become tight and

shiny.
- **Pus or Drainage**: In more advanced cases, there may be pus or other fluid drainage from the affected area.
- **Lymph Node Enlargement**: Swollen and tender lymph nodes (lymphadenopathy) near the site of infection may be palpable.

Laboratory Findings

- **Complete blood count (CBC)**: Leukocytosis may be observed in cases of cellulitis, indicating an inflammatory response.
- **Blood Cultures**: These may be performed to identify the causative bacteria and guide antibiotic treatment if the infection is severe or spreading systemically (febrile).
- **Wound Culture**: In cases where there is an open wound or abscess associated with cellulitis, or no response to antibiotics, a deep culture of the wound may be taken to identify the specific bacteria causing the infection.

Imaging Findings

- **Ultrasound**: It is used to assess the depth of the infection, detect the presence of abscesses, or evaluate the extent of tissue involvement.
- **CT Scan**: It may provide more detailed information about the extent and depth of the infection, helping to differentiate cellulitis from deeper tissue infections or other conditions.

Diagnostic Workup

Overall cellulitis is a clinical diagnosis that considers the physical exam findings delineated above, but additional testing can help identify complicating factors or other co-occurring infections. Blood and wound cultures may be considered when suspecting systemic disease and/or atypical organisms, respectively.

- Indications for blood cultures or wound cultures in the diagnosis:
  - Severe local infection
  - Systemic signs present
  - History of recurrence
  - Failure of initial antibiotics
  - Extremes of age
  - Underlying comorbidities
  - Exposure to a human/animal bites
  - Exposure to water associated injury

Positive cultures can help to guide further evaluation for other co-occurring infections such as osteomyelitis or endocarditis. Usefulness of radiographic imaging in cellulitis is to help identify presence of a drainable abscesses or the presence of underlying osteomyelitis, necrotizing fasciitis, or gas gangrene. If there is any suspicion for one of these other infections, radiographic imaging should not be delayed.

- **Differential Diagnoses to Consider**
  - Erysipelas
  - Deep Venous thrombosis
  - Urticarial or allergic skin reactions (hives)
  - Peripheral vascular disease
  - Insect or spider bites
  - Cutaneous lymphangitis
  - Vasculitis

Treatment

The treatment of cellulitis in a hospital setting is focused on effectively combating the bacterial skin infection.
- Patients admitted for cellulitis typically receive intravenous antibiotics, chosen based on the suspected causative bacteria and local resistance patterns.
- Close monitoring of vital signs, particularly temperature and heart rate, is essential to assess the patient's response to treatment and detect any potential complications.
- Wound care and drainage of abscesses, if present, are important aspects of cellulitis treatment, with sterile techniques being paramount.
- In some cases, consultations with infectious disease specialists or surgeons may be necessary for complex or non-responsive cases.
- Patient education regarding the importance of completing the full course of antibiotics, wound care instructions, and signs of worsening infection is crucial.

Always consider providing empiric coverage for beta-hemolytic streptococcus and methicillin sensitive staph. aureus: the two most common pathogens of cellulitis.

- Indications for parenteral coverage
  - Systemic toxicity
  - Rapid progression or extensive erythema

- o Unable to tolerate oral therapies

  - In the setting of severe sepsis, septic shock, or immunocompromise
    - o Vancomycin or daptomycin

PLUS

    - o Cefepime or meropenem (in suspected ESBL)

  - Indications for MRSA coverage:
    - o Purulent drainage or exudate
    - o Known MRSA colonization or past infection
    - o Recent antibiotic use
    - o Recent healthcare exposure
    - o Intravenous drug use
    - o Purulent drainage

  - Parenteral therapies targeting beta-hemolytic strep and MRSA include
    - o Vancomycin or Daptomycin

  - Parenteral therapies targeting beta-hemolytic strep and MSSA include
    - o Cefazolin, Nafcillin, Oxacillin, or Flucloxacillin
    - o For severe beta-lactam allergy
      - Vancomycin

  - Oral therapies targeting beta-hemolytic strep and MRSA include
    - o Trimethoprim-sulfamethoxazole

or

    - o Amoxicillin PLUS doxycycline

or

    - o Linezolid, or Clindamycin

  - Oral therapies targeting beta-hemolytic strep and MSSA include
    - o Dicloxacillin, Flucloxacillin, Cephalexin, or Cefadroxil
    - o For severe beta-lactam allergy
      - Trimethoprim-sulfamethoxazole double strength, Linezolid, or Clindamycin

  - Oral step-down therapies include
    - o Immunocompromised, without identified pathogen
      - Amoxicillin clavulanate PLUS doxycycline

or

- ▪ Trimethoprim-sulfamethoxazole double strength
  - o Stable, not immunocompromised
    - ▪ Cephalexin, Dicloxacillin, or Flucloxacillin

Oral Therapies		
Amoxicillin	875 mg	q12h
Amoxicillin-clavulanate	875 mg / 125 mg	q12h
Cefadroxil	500 mg or	q12h
	1 gram	q24h
Cephalexin	500 mg	q6h
Clindamycin	450 mg	q8h
Dicloxacillin	500 mg	q6h
Doxycycline	100 mg	q12h
Flucloxacillin	500 - 1000 mg	q6h
	2 grams	q6h
Linezolid	600 mg	q12h
Trimethoprim-sulfamethoxazole	Single strength: 80 mg / 400 mg	q12h
	Double strength: 160 mg / 800 mg	q12h
**All provided doses are for the ADULT patient with NORMAL kidney function. Please refer to your other favorite resource for AKI, ESRD and pediatric dosing. **		

Intravenous Therapies		
Aztreonam	2 grams	q6-8h
Cefazolin	1 - 2 grams	q8h
Cefepime	2 grams	q8h
Daptomycin	4 - 6 mg/kg	q24h
Flucloxacillin	2 grams	q6h
Levofloxacin	750 mg	q24h
Meropenem	1 gram	q8h
Nafcillin	1 - 2 grams	q4h
Oxacillin	1 - 2 grams	q4h
Vancomycin	Loading dose: 20 - 35 mg/kg	Once
	Maintenance dose: 15 - 20 mg/kg	q8-12h

	Adjustments based on trough concentration	
All provided doses are for the ADULT patient with NORMAL kidney function. Evaluating the hospital's antibiogram for antibiotic resistance and understanding institutional protocols is crucial. This knowledge can aid in formulating the best effective treatment, preserving patient safety, and combating the growing challenge of antibiotic resistance.		

The duration of therapy is usually 5-6 days for uncomplicated and up to 14 days in the setting of severe infection, slow response to therapy, or immunosuppression.

Intern Mastery

- **Clinical Documentation**
  - Accurate documentation of the type of cellulitis is important and provides clarity to all providers caring for the patient.
  - Ex: Severe sepsis secondary to left lower extremity purulent cellulitis most likely due to gram positive infection
  - o Assess severity of infection, if patient can be diagnosed under the criteria of sepsis or SIRS
  - o Determine if cellulitis is purulent or non-purulent
  - o If possible causative organism is gram positive or gram negative, being the first one more common.
  - o Specify the location.
  - o Mention if previous history of MSRA or MDRO

- **Monitoring**
  - Continue assessing daily vitals signs and mental status
  - Daily evaluation of erythema expansion or regression. Redness should be demarcated with skin marker to compare from day one and after initiation of antibiotic therapy.
  - CBC and inflammatory markers to determine effectiveness of therapy.
  - Consultation to Infectious disease granted if patient with history of MDRO, multiple or recurrent episodes of cellulitis, immunocompromised patients, no improvement with antibiotic therapy in the next 48 hours. You may also consider a consultation to wound care if debridement or incision and drainage is needed.

- **Discharge Planning**

- Education
    - Keep infected area clean, dry, and elevate often to decrease swelling.
    - Finish antibiotic course as prescribed
    - Mark the boundary of the infected area to track improvement
    - It is normal for area of redness to initially extend beyond the current surface area over first 48 hours, but after 48 hours on treatment the redness should start receding. If it does not, contact your doctor.
- Medications
    - Narrow antibiotics to target the pathogen based on culture and susceptibility profile
    - NSAIDs are not recommended as they can mask serious adverse effects of cellulitis infections
    - Pain management as needed.
- Follow ups
    - Call your doctor in the case of any new onset nausea, vomiting, diarrhea, rash, discharge, fever, worsening pain, swelling or concerning symptoms.

- **Guideline: IDSA practice guidelines for the diagnosis and management of skin and soft tissue infections (2014)**
    - Treatment of predisposing conditions such as edema, obesity, eczema, and venous insufficiency can reduce reoccurrence and improve healing time.
    - Purulent skin and soft tissue infections
        - Obtaining gram stain and culture of pus is recommended, but is not a requirement to start treatment.
        - Incision and drainage should be performed on inflamed epidermoid cysts, carbuncles, abscesses or large furuncles.
        - Antibiotic treatment for MRSA should be administered in cases where prior antibiotic treatments have failed, immunocompromised patients, or in the setting of SIRS and hypotension.
    - Recurrent Skin Abscesses
        - Recurrent abscess should prompt a more in-depth search for other causes such as the presence of a pilonidal cyst, hidradenitis suppurativa, or foreign material in the area. Consider workup for neutrophil disorders may also be warranted.
        - Incision and drainage with repeat cultures should be performed early in the course of infection.

- o If a patient experiences three or more recurrent episodes in a year, prophylactic antibiotics should be considered. Special care should be made to address any predisposing factors. Prophylactic antibiotics can be continued for as long as the predisposing factor persists.
- Erysipelas and Cellulitis
  - o Blood cultures, cultures and microscopic examination of cutaneous aspirates, biopsies, or swabs are only recommended in patients with malignancy on chemotherapy, neutropenia, severe cell-mediated immunodeficiency, immersion injuries, and animal bites.
  - o Simple cellulitis without systemic signs should receive antibiotics against streptococci. Cellulitis with systemic signs of infection, systemic antibiotics are indicated. Coverage against methicillin-susceptible S. aureus (MSSA) is reasonable. Treatment with vancomycin or other antimicrobial effective against both MRSA and streptococci is recommended in the setting of cellulitis associated with penetrating trauma, evidence of MRSA infection elsewhere, nasal colonization with MRSA, injection drug use, or SIRS. In immunocompromised patients, broad-spectrum antibiotics should be used. Vancomycin plus either piperacillin-tazobactam or imipenem/meropenem is reasonable for severe infections.
  - o A 5 days course of antibiotics is the standard, but this can be extended if the infection has not fully resolved within that time.
  - o Patients who do not meet SIRS criteria can be managed on an outpatient basis. Inpatient treatment is only recommended if there is concern for a deeper or necrotizing infection, for patients with poor adherence to therapy, for infection in a severely immunocompromised patient, or if outpatient treatment is failing.
- **ACP appropriate use of short course antibiotics in common infections (2021)**
  - o In the setting of cellulitis, a 5-6-day course of antibiotics that target streptococci is appropriate in the setting of non-purulent cellulitis. However, close PCP follow-up is recommended.

Hospital Course

In the ED, Mr. K. was hypotensive, tachycardia and febrile. CBC was notable for leukocytosis of 16,000. Urinalysis revealed pH of 7.1, positive leukocyte esterase, blood and nitrites and significant white blood cells. Ultrasound of the kidneys was unremarkable, without nephrolithiasis or hydronephrosis. He was started on IV fluids and antibiotics. Once admitted to medicine, urology was consulted given recent TURP. The following day Mr. K did not appropriately respond to therapy as expected, with worsening leukocytosis and flank pain, so a CT abdomen pelvis was ordered which revealed pyelonephritis with perinephric abscess. Upon review of urine cultures, MRDO Klebsiella species was appreciated. Infectious disease was promptly consulted, and the patient was switched to IV meropenem to tailored antibiotic. The patient clinically improved over the next 5 days, and subsequently discharged to SNF on appropriate oral antibiotics and with outpatient urology follow up.

Challenge Questions

1. Erythematous raised lesion on the left side of the face, with distinct margins, tender to palpation and associated with fever, is most consistent with?
   a. Cellulitis
   b. Erysipelas
   c. Impetigo
   d. Herpes zoster

2. After antibiotics and IVF, what is the most appropriate next step in a patient with sepsis secondary to a localized skin abscess:
   a. Add metronidazole
   b. Surgery consult for I&D
   c. Add MRSA coverage
   d. MRI of the affected extremity

3. A young patient, without comorbidities, hemodynamically stable, with non purulent cellulitis of left leg, can be treated as outpatient?
   a. True
   b. False

Chapter IV: Neurology
Authors and Editors

Editors
Luis Daniel Lugo MD MBA
Parker Williams DO MBA

Authors
Dominique Montecino MD
Andrew Rivera MD
Zein Barakat DO MS

Chapter IV: Neurology and Alcohol Withdrawal

Evaluation of a patient with hypertension presenting with "right-arm weakness."

Mrs. H is a 75-year-old female with a PMH of hyperlipidemia, hypertension, chronic kidney disease and type II diabetes mellitus admitted to the emergency department due to a sudden onset of right-sided upper and lower extremity weakness and left-sided facial droop that began 3 hours ago. The patient was accompanied by her husband who stated the patient was having breakfast, when she began having difficulty feeding herself and drooling, followed by progressive weakness of her right side. Her husband endorsed moderate activity level at baseline including cooking and doing crossword puzzles. The patient was recently dismissed from work and has been drinking around a moderate amount of alcohol. Her husband believes that this new pattern is affecting her activities of daily living. She is right-handed. The patients home medications include atorvastatin 40 mg daily, lisinopril 10 mg daily, and metformin 1000 mg twice a day.

On exam, patient appears anxious and tremulous. Her blood pressure on arrival was 155/100 and heart rate was 120 bpm. SpO2 was 96% on room air. Finger stick blood glucose was 128 mg/dl. ECG showed sinus tachycardia with regular rhythm. Computed tomography without contrast of the head was ordered.

HPI Pertinent Positives

- Right hemiparcsis
- Right nasolabial fold ablation
- Hyperglycemia
- Moderate alcohol use

Associated Comorbidities

- Smoking
- Hypertension
- Diabetes mellitus
- Chronic kidney disease

Cerebrovascular Accident

A stroke, also known as a cerebrovascular accident (CVA), is a sudden interruption of blood supply to the brain, leading to brain cell damage or death. Ischemic strokes (most common CVA) result from blocked blood vessels, while hemorrhagic strokes occur due to blood vessel rupture. Unlike a stroke, a TIA, or transient ischemic attack, is marked by a temporary focal neurological impairment without any signs of infarction on neuroimaging. Individuals who experience a TIA are at a heightened risk of stroke within the initial 48 hours after the onset of symptoms and thus should undergo a swift evaluation. Hypertension (high blood pressure) is the single most important modifiable risk factor for strokes. Other risk factors include smoking, diabetes, obesity, atrial fibrillation (AFib), high cholesterol, and a family history of stroke.

Physical Exam

- **Weakness:** Unilateral weakness the arms, legs and or facial weakness without sensory, visual, or cognitive deficits suggest a pure motor stroke secondary to thrombosis or small ICH. Symptoms typically worsen over minutes to hours.
    - o For strokes affecting the anterior circulation, look for abnormalities with language or a combination of unilateral motor and sensory changes.
    - o Conversely, for strokes affecting the posterior circulation, look for changes in vision, hearing, dizziness or bilateral motor or sensory changes.
- A loss of consciousness without focal signs is concerning for subarachnoid hemorrhage (SAH). Other examination findings suggestive of SAH include confusion and somnolence, nuchal rigidity, pupillary dilation from compression of the oculomotor nerve (cranial nerve III) by a posterior communicating artery aneurysm, or subhyaloid hemorrhages on funduscopy.

Laboratory Data

- CBC, Blood glucose, coagulation studies, HDL, LDL and Triglycerides
    - o Hypoglycemia, low blood sugar, may mimic focal neurological deficits, and patients may respond quickly to intervention.

Imaging Findings

- **Non-contrast head CT scan**: Imaging is essential to rule out ischemic vs hemorrhagic or mimicking pathologies (tumors). Before starting treatment for stroke, it is necessary to perform neuroimaging.
- **Brain MRI**: It is more effective in detecting acute infarction compared

to CT, but it is not the preferred initial test for ruling out hemorrhagic stroke or determining thrombolysis treatment decisions for ischemic stroke.

Diagnostic Workup

Patients who have a transient ischemic attack in an area of the brain supplied by an internal carotid artery with over 70% extracranial stenosis are at the highest risk of suffering a stroke. For all individuals experiencing a transient ischemic attack, it's necessary to promptly conduct vascular imaging of the internal carotid artery and perform a cardiac assessment for atrial fibrillation. Carotid ultrasonography is recommended in assessing TIAs and stroke; however, for detecting intracranial large vessel atherosclerosis, magnetic resonance angiography and CT angiography prove to be more sensitive. Atrial fibrillation, being the most prevalent cardioembolic source of stroke, necessitates anticoagulation. Still, the initiation of anticoagulation cannot be justified solely based on radiographic indications of a cardioembolic source. It should be considered to carry out extended cardiac monitoring for numerous patients suffering from embolic stroke of an unknown origin (previously referred to as cryptogenic stroke), as they may have undetected episodes of atrial fibrillation.

Subdural hematomas are most prevalent in the elderly population. The acute symptoms include numbness, weakness, seizures, visual alterations. This hematoma occurs due to tearing of bridging veins between arachnoid and dura mater and presents as a crescent shape appearance on CT w/o contrast. Spontaneous intracerebral hemorrhage are most associated with hypertension and older age. Positive history of drawn-out new onset thunderclap headaches is suggestive. Cerebral amyloid angiopathy is also one of the main causes of recurrent lobar hemorrhage.

- **Differential Diagnoses to Consider**
    - Hypoglycemia
    - Multiple Sclerosis
    - Atypical migraines
    - Metabolic Encephalopathy

Treatment

- **Ischemic Stroke**:
    - Intravenous tissue plasminogen activator (tPA) is a time-sensitive treatment to dissolve clots. Eligible patients should receive tPA within the first 4.5 hours after symptom onset.

- Mechanical thrombectomy may be considered for large vessel occlusions.
- Secondary prevention involves antiplatelet or anticoagulant therapy (as appropriate), blood pressure control, statins, and lifestyle modifications.
    - Blood pressure goals *before* receiving tPA should be SBP < 185 and DBP < 110. Thereafter, BP should be stabilized to SBP <180 and DBP < 105
    - If patient is not a candidate for tPA, BP should not exceed SBP >220 and DBP >120.

- **Hemorrhagic Stroke:**
    - Hemorrhagic strokes often require intensive care and neurosurgical evaluation.
    - Blood pressure control is crucial to prevent rebleeding.

- **Bell's Palsy:**
    - This is a condition characterized by unexplained peripheral facial paralysis. It is believed most cases stem from the reactivation of the herpes simplex virus. Unilateral facial weakness that affects both upper (eye, forehead) and lower (mouth, cheek) muscles might occur, possibly accompanied by taste loss. Initiating treatment early with corticosteroids, for example within days of noticing symptoms, improves the chances of full recovery.

In patients with TIA or minor stroke (NIHSS score of 5 or less) initiating dual antiplatelet therapy (aspirin and clopidogrel) within 24 hours after symptom onset and continuing it for 21 days has proven effective in reducing the risk of recurrent ischemic stroke for up to 90 days from symptom onset.

For a select group of patients showing clinical signs of a **large-vessel occlusion** and specific examination and radiological results, such as discernible neurological impairment and minor yet visible ischemic changes on radiography, **endovascular therapy** can be contemplated within 24 hours of stroke onset. For patients with acute ischemic stroke who are not eligible for either thrombolysis or endovascular stroke therapy, antiplatelet therapy is the mainstay of acute treatment. When given orally or via rectal administration within the first 48 hours following a stroke, Aspirin lessens the immediate risk of another stroke. Its application during the acute phase is considered a fundamental quality-of-care benchmark specific to stroke treatment. The schedule for starting antiplatelet therapy should be meticulously reconsidered in patients who have experienced a hemorrhagic transformation following an ischemic stroke. This is particularly important as the optimal timing can differ based on the severity of the stroke, with some experts suggesting a range from 2 days for minor strokes to up to 12 days for more severe cases.

Stroke rehabilitation, including physical therapy, speech therapy, and occupational therapy, plays a pivotal role in recovery. Early rehabilitation should begin as soon as the patient's medical condition allows. In these patients, consult your hospitals inpatient rehabilitation (PM&R) service.

Secondary Stroke Prevention:
- Aggressively control modifiable risk factors, including blood pressure, diabetes, and smoking cessation.
- Stroke patients should be started on statins, and lifestyle modifications.

Intern Mastery

1. **Clinical Documentation**
   a) Accurate documentation of the type of stroke or Bell's palsy is important and provides clarity to all providers caring for the patient.
   b) Transient Ischemic Attack vs. Acute ischemic stroke vs. Stroke
   c) Acute ischemic stroke secondary to hypertension
   d) Idiopathic Bell's palsy vs. Bell's palsy likely secondary to "x"

1. **Monitoring**
   a) Monitoring a stroke patient with neurochecks is crucial to promptly detect any neurological deterioration, thus enabling immediate intervention. According to research published in the American Heart Association journal, the role of neurochecks is to quickly identify any neurological changes in patients recently hospitalized due to stroke.
      - Ensuring aspiration and fall precautions is also essential. Aspiration can lead to pneumonia, a common complication after stroke, while falls can result in further injury. The American Heart Association recommends routine dysphagia screening before the patient starts eating, drinking, or receiving oral medications to prevent aspiration.
      - Consult the inpatient rehabilitation (PM&R) service as needed. Fall precautions, including regular assessments of gait and balance, the use of assistive devices as needed, and

environmental modifications, can significantly reduce the risk of falls.

- Unless there are high-risk stroke characteristics, such as stenosis exceeding 70% or fast-paced progression of stenosis, routine revascularization of the internal carotid artery is not typically recommended for primary prevention of stroke.

1. **Discharge Planning**
   a) Several considerations should be made based on evidence-based guidelines from the American Heart Association (AHA).
      - Firstly, it's important to assess the patient's rehabilitation needs. This involves evaluating their physical, cognitive, and emotional status and determining the need for therapies such as occupational, speech, and physical therapy.
      - Secondly, ensuring the initiation of appropriate medical therapies is crucial. Antiplatelet therapy is recommended for patients with ischemic stroke or transient ischemic attack (TIA), as it helps prevent recurrent strokes. Statin therapy is also advised for patients with atherosclerotic ischemic stroke or TIA.
      - Thirdly, coordinating follow-up care is essential. This includes scheduling follow-up visits and providing clear instructions regarding medication management, lifestyle modifications, and recognition of stroke symptoms. Patient education should be prioritized. Informing patients and their families about the nature of the condition, the purpose and side effects of prescribed medications, the importance of adherence to treatment, and strategies to reduce risk factors can improve outcomes.

1. **Clinical Guideline from the American Heart Association**
   a) In patients who have experienced a transient ischemic attack, adding clopidogrel to aspirin for 21 days has been shown to be effective in reducing the risk for subsequent stroke compared with monotherapy with either agent alone. In patients treated with dual antiplatelet therapy following a transient ischemic attack or minor stroke, aspirin should be continued following discontinuation of clopidogrel at 21 days.
      - In patients with acute stroke or TIA, direct oral anticoagulants have not been established as effective at reducing the risk for subsequent adverse outcomes.

Challenge Questions

1. What do all patients with stroke or TIA require:
    - Emergent head CT without contrast (to rule out intracranial hemorrhage), ECG and telemetry (to rule out AF), duplex ultrasonography of internal carotid artery; MRA and CTA are appropriate confirmatory tests and an echocardiography (to rule out LV or valvular thrombus).

2. Regular screening for thrombophilia or investigation with TEE is not recommended for patients who have experienced a Transient Ischemic Attack (TIA) or stroke.
    a. **True**
    b. False

3. When is early carotid revascularization recommended after a nondisabling stroke?
    - Early carotid revascularization is recommended after a nondisabling stroke or TIA if ipsilateral carotid stenosis is >50%, provided the patient is likely to live 5 years.

Alcohol Withdrawal

Excessive alcohol consumption is a significant health concern in the United States, ranking as the fourth leading cause of preventable death source. The U.S. Preventive Services Task Force (USPSTF) advises regular screening for unhealthy alcohol use. Suggested screening tools encompass the Alcohol Use Disorders Identification Test (AUDIT), the abbreviated AUDIT-Consumption (AUDIT-C), and a single-question screen asking about the frequency of heavy drinking episodes in the past year.

Following a positive screening result, an assessment for alcohol use disorder should be conducted. This evaluation should also include the severity of the disorder, any related health consequences like hepatic, cardiac, and neurologic sequelae, and any potential comorbid psychiatric, chronic pain, and substance use disorders that might necessitate interdisciplinary treatment and subspecialty referral.

Treatment plans should be individualized according to the patient's risk level and may consist of psychotherapy, such as cognitive behavioral therapy (CBT), and pharmacotherapy. Alcohol withdrawal is a common complication of alcohol use disorder.

Physical Exam

- **Early Autonomic Symptoms**: Symptoms such as tremulousness, diaphoresis, and palpitations can manifest 6 hours following the last alcohol consumption.
    - Alcoholic hallucinosis, characterized by hallucinations without sensorium clouding, typically occurs 12 to 24 hours after alcohol cessation. Withdrawal seizures may happen between 12 to 48 hours after stopping alcohol use.
- **Delirium tremens (DT)**: 48 to 96 hours post the last alcoholic drink, is characterized by vivid autonomic activation (like hypertension, tachycardia) and altered mental state. It is often preceded by mild withdrawal symptoms or withdrawal seizures. In a meta-analysis, autonomic disarray with diastolic hypertension was found to be an early potential sign for impending DT.

Laboratory Data

- Elevated MCV
- An elevated γ-glutamyltransferase level, AST-ALT ratio >2 are all suggestive but not diagnostic of alcohol use disorder.

Diagnostic Workup

The diagnostic workup for a patient with suspected alcohol withdrawal typically involves obtaining a detailed history of the patient's alcohol use, such as the quantity and frequency of consumption, and when the last drink was consumed. Any previous experiences with withdrawal symptoms or treatments should also be documented. The physician should also do a thorough physical examination to identify signs of alcohol withdrawal like tremors, increased heart rate, sweating, nausea, or vomiting. Look for signs of chronic alcohol abuse such as liver disease, malnutrition, or neurological issues. Conduct a mental health evaluation to identify any comorbid psychiatric conditions like depression, anxiety, or psychosis which are common in individuals with alcohol use disorders.

Validate your working diagnosis with tools like the Alcohol Use Disorders Identification Test (AUDIT) or the Clinical Institute Withdrawal Assessment for Alcohol, Revised (CIWA-Ar) to assess the severity of alcohol withdrawal. Lab tests to consider include a complete blood count (CBC), liver function tests, electrolytes, blood alcohol level, and a urine toxicology screen. These tests can help identify alcohol-related health complications and rule out other causes for the patient's symptoms.

Use the Prediction of Alcohol Withdrawal Severity Scale (PAWSS) to predict the likelihood of severe withdrawal syndrome.

- **Differential Diagnoses to Consider**
  - Hypoglycemia
  - Drug induced psychosis
  - Opioid Withdrawal
  - Thyrotoxicosis
  - Neuroleptic Malignant Syndrome

Treatment

The USPSTF suggests that individuals with alcohol use disorder should be referred for specialized treatment.

- Naltrexone, a medication used to prevent relapse in alcohol abuse and dependence, can be administered even to patients who are still actively drinking. However, it is not suitable for patients on or withdrawing from opioids, or those with liver failure or hepatitis.
- Disulfiram, a second-line treatment, leads to acetaldehyde buildup if alcohol is consumed, causing symptoms like flushing, headaches, vomiting, and necessitates complete avoidance of any alcohol-containing items.

Patients with moderate to severe alcohol withdrawal symptoms, or other significant reasons, might require hospitalization. Hospitalized patients are typically prescribed benzodiazepines (lorazepam), especially if they have a history of alcohol-related seizures or delirium tremens, exhibit significant withdrawal symptoms, are pregnant, or have acute medical or surgical conditions. Long-acting benzodiazepines are usually favored. A symptom-triggered regimen, such as the Clinical Institute Withdrawal Assessment for Alcohol, Revised (CIWA), is commonly employed to manage alcohol withdrawal. Adjunctive therapies like β-blockers and clonidine may help manage tachycardia and hypertension, but they are not used as standalone treatments.

Intern Mastery

- **Clinical Documentation**
  - Accurate documentation of the alcohol withdrawal is important and provides clarity to all providers caring for the patient.
  - Alcohol Withdrawal Syndrome with DT vs. Alcohol intoxication
  - Alcohol use disorder vs. Elevated alcohol level

- **Monitoring**
  - Vital signs
    - o Patients progressing toward DT may demonstrate worsening changes in their vital signs. Monitor them closely.
    - o Assess the total number in the CIWA scale. This number should correlate with the patient's improvement and further need for benzodiazepine. Downtitrate benzodiazepines as needed. Not all patients who stop alcohol abruptly experience withdrawal, and treatment with benzodiazepines is not always needed.
    - o Administer thiamine replacement prior to giving glucose and refrain from using antipsychotic medications, as they could potentially disrupt and reduce the patient's seizure threshold.
    - o In patient's with thrombocytopenia, consider long-standing alcohol use and an right-upper quadrant ultrasound.

- **Discharge planning**
  - Education: Upon being discharged, patients with alcohol use disorder or those recovering from alcohol withdrawal should receive a comprehensive treatment plan to help maintain their sobriety and prevent relapse. This plan should include ongoing outpatient therapy, either individual or group, and may involve family members for support. The use of medications such as naltrexone, acamprosate, or disulfiram may be recommended, depending on the patient's specific needs and conditions. It is also crucial that these patients continue to abstain from alcohol consumption, as even small amounts can trigger a relapse.
    - o Connect the patient with community resources that can offer further support, such as Alcoholics Anonymous or other peer support groups.
    - o Regular follow-up appointments with a healthcare provider should be scheduled to monitor the patient's progress and adjust treatment as necessary. Patients should also be educated about the signs of a potential relapse and advised to seek immediate medical attention if these occur.
    - o Lifestyle modifications, such as stress management techniques and healthy eating habits, can also play a significant role in recovery and should be encouraged.

- **2020-2025 Dietary Guidelines for Americans:** Adults of legal drinking age can choose not to drink, or to drink in moderation by limiting intake to 2 drinks or less in a day for men or 1 drink or less in a day for women, on days when alcohol is consumed.

Challenge Questions

1. What should be administered prior to any glucose load in patients admitted with alcohol intoxication?
   a. Intravenous fructose
   b. Intravenous magnesium
   c. **Vitamin B1**
   d. Vitamin B12

2. Benzodiazepines should be carefully titrated in which of the following patients:
   a. Bradycardia
   b. **Hepatic impairment**
   c. Hypertension
   d. A and B

3. Which of the following is associated with optic neuritis?
   a. Naltrexone
   b. Acamprosate
   c. **Disulfiram**
   d. Gabapentin

Hospital Course

This patients CT scan showed hypoattenuation in the basal ganglia, with loss of gray-white matter interface concerning for an ischemic stroke in the basal ganglia. Further work-up was unremarkable for a large-vessel occlusion and the patient did not require reperfusion therapy. The patient was started on aspirin, stated and admitted to the medicine floor under CIWA protocol with close neurochecks.

Chapter V: Gastroenterology and Oncology

Authors and Editors

Editors
Luis Daniel Lugo MD MBA
Parker Williams DO MBA

Authors
Daniela Carralero Somoza MD
Joshua Tsai MD MBA
Christiane Martell Rodriguez MD
Michael Sabina DO

Chapter V: Gastroenterology and Oncology

Evaluation of a patient with "coughing up blood"

A 57-year-old male with a past medical history of hypertension and type 2 diabetes mellitus came into the emergency room with multiple chief complaints including blood-stained bed sheets. He endorsed a four-month history of chronic right-sided thoracic and epigastric pain that recently worsened over the past 48 hours and a one-week history of black, tarry stools, and several episodes of vomiting with tinges of blood that were associated with nausea. The nausea and vomiting prevented him from taking his home medications. He has been progressively short of breath and fatigued. He stated that he's uninsured, which is why he prolonged visiting the doctor.

The patient's home medications include amlodipine 5 mg daily (QD), metformin 1000 mg twice a day (BID), ibuprofen 800 mg three times a day (TID), and aspirin 325 mg QD. He stated that he has been obtaining these medications from third-party sources within the United States and his home country of Mexico. He had been taking the ibuprofen and aspirin in conjunction for the past several months because of the worsening pain that has been waking him up at night. His stools have become darker with a "coffee ground-like" color. He also endorses increasing nausea and bouts of vomiting that have been more forceful lately. His pain was initially relieved by over-the-counter ibuprofen and acetaminophen, but it has since become resistant to the medications. He denied any trauma to the area or recent change in his physical activity or sleep hygiene. Regarding social history, the patient stated that he smoked cigarettes during his twenties for about two years. He also worked in the construction field for 30 years that required him to lay insulation in newly constructed homes. He denied alcohol abuse and illicit drug use. Upon further questioning, he reported a history of GERD for which he usually takes OTC calcium carbonate tablets.

In the emergency department, his labs were found to be significant for a Hb of 9.9, Hct 29.9%., MCV 75.5, and a WBC of 13.8. Chest x-ray and chest CT scan were performed and revealed a 3 cm spiculated nodule in the periphery of the right upper lobe and air under diaphragm.

HPI Pertinent Positives

- Fatigue
- Shortness of breath
- Melena

- Blood-tinged sputum
- Chronic back pain
- NSAID abuse
- Sharp epigastric pain
- History of smoking
- Chronic right-sided thoracic back pain
- Construction insulation work

Associated Comorbidities

- NSAIDs use abuse.
- Hypertension
- Diabetes Mellitus Type 2

Upper Gastrointestinal Bleed

Upper gastrointestinal bleed can be caused by peptic ulcers, gastritis, varices, esophagitis, or esophageal tears. Signs of upper gastrointestinal tract bleeding can range from hematemesis to melena.

Perforated peptic ulcer disease is a serious medical condition. A perforated peptic ulcer occurs when there is a rupture of the gastric mucosa or the duodenum due to an untreated peptic ulcer. This allows gastric acid or intestinal fluids to leak into the abdominal cavity. Patients with perforated peptic ulcer typically experience sudden, abdominal pain that may be referred to the chest, back or shoulder. Patients typically engage in guarding, suffer from abdominal tenderness, and can present with signs of peritonitis, such as fever and tachycardia. Types of peptic ulcer vary by location. Duodenal ulcers typically cause patients to feel pain relief with eating but experience pain between meals, especially at night. In contrast to gastric ulcers.

Risk factors include infection with H. pylori, history of peptic ulcers, smoking, alcohol use, and NSAIDs use. The incidence of perforated peptic ulcer disease has decreased over the years due to improved treatment of peptic ulcers with medication like PPIs and the eradication of H. Pylori infections.

The prognosis of upper GI bleed depends on the severity of the bleeding and the underlying disease. Mild cases may resolve with supportive care while more severe bleeds might require not only medical but also surgical interventions. The mortality rate has improved thanks to medical advancements and is strictly correlated to the onset of symptoms, the timeliness of seeking medical care and the timely and adequate diagnosis and management of the patient's condition. The risk of recurrence is influenced by the cause of the GI bleed. Patients with peptic ulcer are at higher risk of recurrence if H. pylori is not treated or if NSAID use is not stopped. Same goes with esophageal varices, tears and gastritis. If the culprit and primary risk is not diminished (example: alcohol cessation, tobacco cessation, continuous vomiting) the risk of occurrence increases.

Physical Exam

- **Blood pressure**: can be decreased due to blood loss, or in early signs can be increased due to pain.
- **Heart rate**: generally increased due to blood loss, as a sign of peritonitis, or pain itself.
- **Respiratory Rate:** can be normal or increased as trying to compensate for presence of metabolic acidosis or pain itself. Hypoventilation if patient is in too much distress that they had stopped respiratory effort and have started to breathe slowly.
- **Temperature:** fever can be present as a sign of peritonitis.
- **General appearance:** pale, sweaty, hunched-over posture to minimize pain.
- **Skin:** decreased skin turgor, dry.
- **HEENT**: Mouth examination can have residual blood from blood in vomit.
- **Cardiovascular:** tachycardia.
- **Pulmonary:** typically, normal breath sounds, crackles can be heard if aspiration has occurred, tachypnea might be present due to pain or compensation for metabolic/respiratory imbalances.
- **Abdominal examination:** tenderness to the touch, guarding and rigidity, rebound tenderness, distended abdomen (can look swollen or bloated), decreased or absent bowel sounds (may indicate paralytic ileus).

Laboratory Data

- **Complete Blood Count (CBC)**:
  - Anemia due to blood loss
  - Slight leukocytosis but not always present (may suggest peritonitis).
- **Comprehensive Metabolic Panel (CMP)**:
  - Decreased potassium due to gastrointestinal losses
  - Hyponatremia due to vomiting or fluid loss.

- BUN and Creatinine may be normal or increased if there is decreased blood flow and AKI is present.
- Hyperglycemia due to stress
- Elevated lactic acid from leakage of GI contents and ischemia
- **Arterial blood gases (may vary on severity of perforation):**
  - Metabolic acidosis: accumulation of lactic acid and other metabolic byproducts from perforation and leakage.
  - Metabolic alkalosis: if extensive vomiting that caused too much loss of HCL
  - Respiratory Acidosis: due to hypoventilation in the setting of being present.
  - Base excess: negative, indicating possible metabolic acidosis.

Imaging Findings

- **Abdominal XRAY** [lateral decubitus preferable] if CT not available
  - Free air in abdomen (air under diaphragm)
- **CT Scan**
  - Intraperitoneal fluid, pneumoperitoneum, bowel wall thickening, mesenteric fat streaking
  - With contrast: Presence of extraluminal water-soluble contrast
- **POCUS**
  - Air under abdominal fascia

Diagnostic Workup

The main approach of the diagnosis of acute upper gastrointestinal bleeding is a thorough history and physical examination of the patient. Important medical information includes medical history, all the medications that the patient is currently taking, social history including alcohol or tobacco use. It is important to ask about any recent procedures or intervention. This information can help guide further diagnostic test and treatment options.

The gold standard diagnostic tool of suspected upper GI bleeding is endoscopy which allows direct visualization of the esophagus, stomach, and duodenum. If only melena is seen and upper endoscopy is unrevealing, a colonoscopy can be performed in most cases. In cases with contraindications to endoscopy or negative upper and lower endoscopy, nuclear medicine scans, CT angiography, or swallowed video capsule endoscopy (miniature camera for direct visual and diagnostic evaluation) can be performed.

- **Differential Diagnoses to Consider**
  - Peptic Ulcer +/- Perforation
  - Erosive gastritis
  - Esophageal varices
  - Mallory- Weiss Tear +/- Boerhaave's

Treatment

General management will always aim to hemodynamically stabilize the patient, protect the airway, aid in pain control and investigate for the cause in order to prevent further damage. The first step is to assess the patient vital signs, protect the airway, volume resuscitation and start with basic management which includes keeping the patient NPO, insert 2 large-bore IVs. Further actions include laboratory to assess hemoglobin levels, platelet count, coagulation profile, renal and liver function.

Treatment strategies vary depending on the cause and severity of bleeding. If patient is hemodynamically stable, conservative management such as IV fluids, blood transfusions and later on lifestyle modifications may be sufficient.

We should be able to identify when the patient is in shock even before taking the history or sending labs. You should be able to identify threatening situations just by looking at the vital signs. If the patient presents with severe hypotension and tachycardia. You should have an adequate peripheral access to begin with fluid resuscitation. IVFs should be given in boluses of 500-1000 ml over less than 30 min. This first step in unstable patients should not be delayed. At the moment there is not a correct answer for which type of IV fluid you can choose. In some hospitals normal saline is used and in other lactated ringers is preferred. Keep in mind that these patients may need to be transferred to ICU for close monitoring.

If you suspected that the patient is actively bleeding and having hypovolemia, you should not wait for labs to come back. You may start the transfusion guided by hemodynamic conditions. If hemoglobin comes back below 7 g/dl you should start with transfusion as well.

All patients are managed with proton pump inhibitors and endoscopy regardless of whether the patient being stable or not.

- **Peptic ulcer Disease**
  - If H. pylori is positive, the recommended treatment is:

- Clarithromycin triple therapy: PPI twice a day, Clarithromycin twice a day and Amoxicillin twice a day or Metronidazole 3 times daily, or,
- Bismuth quadruple therapy: PPI twice a day, bismuth four times daily, metronidazole 4 times daily or tetracyclines four times daily

- **Erosive Gastritis**
  - Avoid the offensive agents such as NSAIDS, alcohol, stress, drugs
  - Treat the infection.
  - PPI for 4-8 weeks
  - If the patient requires aspirin or NSAIDS you can prescribe PPI as maintenance therapy.

- **Esophageal Varices**
  - Start Beta-blocker, if contraindicated use nitrates as alternative
  - (decrease portal pressures)
  - IV Octreotide *(dose?)*
  - Endoscopic band ligation
  - TIPS (Transjugular intrahepatic portosystemic shunt) if above methods fail

- **Mallory- Weiss Tear**
  - Proton Pump Inhibitors, Antiemetics such as ondansetron or metoclopramide
  - Patient with active bleeding can be treated with epinephrine local injection (reduce the bleeding through vasoconstriction) and thermoregulation.
  - If treatment above fail choose embolization of the artery

Intern Mastery

- **Clinical Documentation**
  - Accurate documentation of the type of gastrointestinal bleeding is important and provides clarity to all providers caring for the patient.
  - Acute upper gastrointestinal bleeding secondary to peptic ulcer perforation on chronic NSAID use
  - Anemia secondary to blood loss from upper gastrointestinal bleed
  - Metabolic acidosis secondary to peptic ulcer perforation
  - AKI secondary to blood loss

- **Monitoring**
  - Vital signs
    - o Monitor blood pressure in case patient becomes

hypotensive due to blood loss.
- Hemoglobin and Hematocrit
  - The initial hemoglobin level in patients with acute upper GI bleeding may be at the patient's baseline because of blood and plasma loss.
  - Remember to send the blood for type and screen.
  - In general, the goal is to maintain hemoglobin level > 7 g/dl unless the patient has coronary artery disease or acute coronary symptoms threshold will be > 8 g/dl. We need to make the decisions based on patient's comorbid conditions.
- Platelets
  - If presents with < 50,000, we should proceed with transfusion.
  - If patient is receiving antiplatelet or anticoagulation medications due to ACS or other heart conditions, we may need to place a Cardiology Consult.

- **Discharge planning**
  - Education
    - Educating patients about the common risk factors. Reducing smoking and tobacco consumption. Advise on chronic NSAID use. Encourage questions and shared decision making.
      - Look out for concerning symptoms like melena, hematochezia, hematemesis, loss of appetite, abdominal pain, dizziness, fainting. Importance of seeking medical care on time. If GERD symptoms, abdominal pain, heartburn arise.
      - Counseling on visiting PCP to further investigate for H. Pylori infection and treat accordingly.
      - Consider proton pump inhibitor for six weeks.
  - Social worker planning if patient has difficulty following up with medical providers or has lack of access to healthcare setting or medication.
  - Counsel on appropriate diet that is not gastro erosive. Limit citric, tomatoes, coffee, teas, chocolate, spices and other harmful gastric food.
  - Patient to call primary care provider if new or worsening symptoms.
    - If concerning symptoms like those mentioned above, visit the Emergency Department.
  - Follow up with primary care physician to establish care and follow

up on screening tests and diagnostic tests if symptoms arise. Stress the importance of following up in order to meet successful treatment plan and adhere to monitoring and refills of medication. Follow up with gastroenterology outpatient to continue medical treatment or any other management can be appropriate.

- **Guideline from the** ACG (American College of Gastroenterology) guidelines 2021 suggest that patients admitted to or under observation in hospital for UGIB undergo endoscopy within 24 hours of presentation
  o Suggest a restrictive policy of red blood cell (RBC) transfusion with a threshold for transfusion at a hemoglobin of 7 g/dL for patients with an upper GI bleed
- AFP (American Family Physician) guidelines 2020
  o Recommends initiation of proton pump inhibitor should not be delayed before endoscopy upon presentation with upper gastrointestinal bleeding.
  o Oral PPI can be used because there was not difference between oral and intravenous PPI in regard to recurrent bleeding, surgery or mortality.

Challenge Questions

1. How may we distinguish upper gastrointestinal bleeding from lower intestinal bleeding? Why is anatomy important to answering this question?
   a. Upper GI bleed typically presents with hematemesis and melena. Lower GI bleed will most likely present with hematochezia. Ligament of Treitz divides the upper and lower GI.

2. Why might Upper GI bleed patient present with an elevated BUN?
   a. Upper GI bleeding can cause prerenal azotemia causing an elevation of BUN. When we have blood loss, we can developed hypotension and subsequently decrease perfusion to the kidney resulting in an elevated BUN.

Lung Adenocarcinoma

Lung adenocarcinoma is characterized as a non-small cell lung cancer and is the most common primary lung cancer among smokers and nonsmokers. It is more commonly found in women and nonsmokers. Adenocarcinoma of the lung is generally seen in the periphery of the lung tissue; however, it can be seen in any location of the lung in practice. The prognosis of non-small cell lung cancer, such as lung adenocarcinoma is typically better because it is more treatable. Those with advanced forms of this malignancy are encouraged to be tested for several tumor markers such as epidermal growth factor receptor (EGFR), thyroid transcription factor-1 (TTF-1) and anaplastic lymphoma kinase (ALK).

There are several subtypes of lung adenocarcinoma such as minimally invasive, invasive non-mucinous, invasive mucinous, colloid, and fetal adenocarcinoma.

Physical Exam

- **Vitals**: Depending on extent of pleural effusions or respiratory compromise from tumor, can be hypoxic with tachypnea and tachycardic. Blood pressure usually stable.
- **General**: Mostly asymptomatic, but in advanced disease can present with appearing distressed secondary to respiratory failure.
- **Pulmonary:** Decreased breath sounds. Lungs clear to auscultation, no wheezes, crackles, rhonchi. Can have pleural effusions, will hear crackles.
- **Cardiovascular:** RRR, no murmurs, rubs, gallops. Can be tachycardic.
- **Abdomen:** Normal bowel sounds, soft, non-distended, no guarding, no rebound tenderness
- **Extremities:** can present with hypertrophic osteoarthropathy
- **HEENT:** Moist mucous membranes,
- **Neuro:** Normal neurological exam

Laboratory Data

- **Complete blood count (CBC):**
  - o   Anemia
  - o   Neutropenia
- **Comprehensive Metabolic Panel (CMP):**
  - o   Hypercalcemia
  - o   Elevated alkaline phosphatase
- Immunochemistry
- Positive expression of napsin A and TTF-1

Imaging Findings

- **Chest X-ray**
  - Although not typically part of the cancer workup, usage of a

chest x-ray can serve as a sensitive imaging modality.

- **CT (computed tomography) Chest with IV contrast**
  - Should be performed in every patient when suspecting some form of lung malignancy.
  - Usage of IV contrast enhances visualization of masses and further tumor involvement. For those with acute kidney injury and/or are at risk of contrast-induced nephropathy, adjunct administration of IV fluids is preferred over CT scans without contrast.
- **Histology**
  - Positive for intracytoplasmic mucin staining and neoplastic glandular appearance.
- **Brain MRI**
  - To assess for metastasis.
- **Bone Scan**
  - If metastasis is suspected.

Diagnostic Workup

The first step to perform whenever lung cancer is suspected, comparison of previous imaging should be performed, whether it be via x-ray or chest CT scan. If previous imaging is not attainable, then a CT scan of the chest should be performed to assess malignancy risk and rule out other differentials like pneumonia.

CT nodules should be radiographically assessed to determine risk and possible need for biopsy. Lung nodules are considered low risk of the size is less then 0.8 cm, the margin of the nodule is smooth, and if the patient is a non-smoker. Intermediate risk is characterized as a nodule size of 0.8 to 2 cm, scalloped margins, and the patient being a current smoker. High risk nodules are defined as a nodule size greater than 2 cm with a spiculated or corona radiata appearance, and the patient being a current smoker.

Nodules that are high risk should undergo surgical excision, and pathology can be determined after the surgery. If a nodule is considered intermediate or low risk, the nodule size is then reassessed. If the size is greater than or equal to 0.8 cm, a PET scan or biopsy should be performed. If the results are suspicious for malignancy, then the nodule should be surgically excised. If it is not suspicious, then serial CT scans of the chest for 2 to 3 years are recommended. If the nodule is 0.5 to 0.7 cm, serial CT scans of the chest should be performed for 2 to 3 years. If the nodule size is less than or equal to 0.4 cm, the provider was the option to either reassure the patient and perform watchful waiting or recommend serial CT scans.

Biopsies are required to confirm the diagnosis of a specific lung malignancy. There are several methods of obtaining the biopsy, depending on the location of the mass. If centrally located, a bronchoscopy with endoscopic transbronchial biopsy using ultrasound can be performed. If peripherally located, needle aspiration via endobronchial CT or ultrasound should be performed by interventional radiology. In the event the cancer is associated with a pleural effusion, a thoracentesis should be performed. Peripherally located pulmonary lesions can also be excised via surgical biopsy can also be performed for both diagnostic and curative purposes. If metastatic disease is suspected, full body imaging including brain imaging and a PET scan should be considered.

If a nodule should be surgically excised, it is important to take into consideration of possible contraindications. Such contraindications include superior vena cava syndrome, supraclavicular node metastasis, scalene node metastasis, tracheal carina involvement, oat cell carcinoma, abnormal pulmonary function testing, myocardial infarction, and metastatic disease.

Staging for NSCLC (non-small cell lung cancer) is performed via the TNM method. T characterizes the primary tumor, N for regional lymph node involvement, and M for distant metastasis.

Lung Adenocarcinoma – final diagnosis is confirmed via pathology and histologic findings. Prior to obtaining the biopsy, imaging via the gold standard of contrast-enhanced CT scan of the chest is performed. Chest CT can also provide information required for the TNM staging method.

- **Differential Diagnoses to Consider**
    - Squamous cell carcinoma given remote smoking history.
    - Pancoast tumor, however, the patient did not present with symptoms significant for superior vena cava syndrome.
    - Vertebral compression fracture however MRI was negative for fractures. Also, the patient did not present with any focal neurologic deficits.
    - Muscle strain, however, the patient did not endorse any extraneous physical activity or improper sleeping positions.
    - Metastatic lesion: Primary cancers can spread to lungs and appear as primary lung disease.
    - Pneumonia: Elevated WBC, febrile, acutely sick
    - Granuloma
    - Benign lung lesions

Treatment

Surgical resection is best treatment for long term survival. Chemoradiotherapy with possible immunotherapy for non resectable cancers. Palliative therapy may also be an option for late-stage patients, without diminishing quality of life.

Intern Mastery

- **Clinical Documentation**
    - Accurate documentation of the type of adenocarcinoma is important and provides clarity to all providers caring for the patient.
    - Lung nodule (benign vs malignant)
    - Non-small cell lung cancer vs small cell lung cancer
    - Primary Lung adenocarcinoma with no metastases
    - Primary Lung adenocarcinoma with metastatic lesions in brain/bone
    - Stage I, II, IIIa, IIIb, IV Lung adenocarcinoma

- **Monitoring**
    - In hospital monitoring
        - Respiratory effort and saturation. Possible supplemental oxygen if patient saturation drops below 92%.
    - Surveillance with CT chest every 6-12 months for two years and annual low dose CT after treatment.
    - Monitoring treatment response
        - Non-genotype driven therapy.
            - Assess after 2 to 3 cycles of systemic therapy via CT scan.
            - PET scans are not recommended due to high sensitivity and low specificity.
            - RECIST 1.1 (response evaluation criteria in solid tumors) when using immunotherapy involving checkpoint inhibitors.
        - Genotype-driven therapy.
            - Assess after 8-12 weeks of genotype-driven therapy via CT scan.
            - PET scans are also not recommended due to the same reasons.
            - Refer to RECIST as noted in the non-

- genotype driven therapy.
- Monitoring after curative-intended treatment
  - ESMO 2021 guidelines:
    - Outpatient visits every six months for the first two years, which includes a CT scan with contrast of the chest and abdomen at the 1- and 2-year checkpoints.
  - ASCO (American Society of Clinical Oncology) 2020 guidelines:
    - Chest CT with contrast of the chest and abdomen every six months for the first two years.
  - ACCP 2013 guidelines:
    - Use physician-based clinical decision making to determine the follow-up and surveillance.
- Monitoring after palliative therapy
  - ESMO 2022 guidelines
    - Chest CT every 3-4 months after using immunotherapy involving checkpoint inhibitors.
    - If an option for continued therapy exists, follow up every six to twelve weeks.
- Routine labs involving CBC and BMP should be obtained.

- **Discharge Planning**
  - **Education**
    - Education regarding the pathology and maintenance to be provided to the patient and family members.
    - Smoking cessation counseling
    - Diet – diets rich in vegetables and fruits that do not contain starch may reduce the risk of lung cancer and further cancer progression; limiting consumption of red meats also help.
    - Goals of care discussion with patient and family.
  - **Medications**
    - Chemotherapy and immunotherapy to be continued outpatient.
  - **Follow Up**
    - Referral to surgical oncology for patients with stage I to stage IIIA for lobectomy or pneumonectomy.
    - Referral to Medical/Radiation oncology for patients who are not surgical candidates.
    - Referral to palliative/hospice or spiritual resources for

those who are not candidates for treatment or those who prefer end-of-life measures.

- **Clinical Guidelines**
  - USPSTF 2021 guidelines
    - An annual low-dose CT scan of adults aged 50 to 80 years of age is recommended for those who have a 20-pack year history and currently smoke, or those who have quit within the past 15 years.
    - Those who have not smoked for 15 years, or those who develop a condition that prevents curative therapy, are no longer indicated to receive this screening measure.
  - ACCP (American College of Chest Physicians) 2021 guidelines
    - Annual screening via low-dose CT in asymptomatic individuals 55 to 77 years of age with a greater than 30-pack-year smoking history and are either continuing to smoke or have quit within the past 15 years
  - Treatment guidelines
    - NIH National Cancer Institute – Non-Small Cell Lung Cancer Treatment (PDQ) 2/17/23
      - Occult – Surgery
      - Stage 0 – Surgery
      - Stage IA and IB – Surgery or adjuvant therapy or radiation therapy
      - Stage IIA and IIB – Surgery with or without adjuvant or neoadjuvant therapy
      - Stage IIIA
        - Resectable disease – Surgery with neoadjuvant or adjuvant therapy
        - Unresectable – Radiation therapy
        - Invades chest wall – Surgery with or without radiation.
      - Stage IIIB – Sequential or concurrent chemotherapy and radiation therapy
      - Newly Diagnosed Stage IV, Relapsed, and Recurrent NSCLC
        - ROS1 inhibitors, NTRK inhibitors, RET inhibitors, MET inhibitors, immune checkpoint inhibitors with or without chemotherapy.

- Progressive Stage IV, relapsed, and recurrent
  - Chemotherapy, EGFR directed therapy, ALK directed TKI's, BRAF V600 and MEK inhibitors, ROS1-directed therapy, NTRK inhibitors, RET inhibitors, MET inhibitors, KRAS G12C inhibitors, HER2-targeted therapy, immunotherapy.

Surgical treatment is the best choice for long term survival and cure in patients with resectable lung cancer. Stage I or II non-small cell lung cancer should be treated with complete surgical resection whenever possible, if not candidates, radiation therapy would be second line treatment. In patients with stage III disease prior to therapy, combined approach using chemoradiotherapy and immunotherapy subsequently if there has been no progression. Surgery can still have a role in these patients with T3 or T4 lesions as long as no spread to mediastinal lymph nodes. Stage IIIB patients are tested for EGFR and ALK mutations. Treatment with tyrosine kinase inhibitors and ALK inhibitors are the treatment for each mutation respectively. If both mutations negative, first line therapy is platinum-based doublet with bevacizumab as possible third agent. Stage IV patients are treated with palliative systemic therapy, immunotherapy, or symptom-based treatment. The goal being to prolong survival without sacrificing quality of life. Some patients will require placement of tunneled pleural catheter for self-controlled drainage in cases of recurrent symptomatic pleural effusions due to malignancy.

Hospital Course

On admission vital signs were significant for blood pressure 95/60, heart rate 112, RR 21, and O2 97% on room air. Physical exam is remarkable for tenderness in the upper quadrant abdomen. Subsequently laboratory test was significant for Hgb levels of 9.0 g/dl, recent baseline was 14 g/dl, coagulation profile was normal and BUN creatinine ratio was 33. These findings along with medical history positive for black tarry stools and hematemesis in the settings of use NSAIDS and aspirin for back pain. Patient was placed 2 IV large bores and 2L of lactated ringer was given. In addition, patient was given a high dose of PPI, and the gastroenterologist was consulted for endoscopy. The source of bleeding was identified in the upper gastrointestinal system and treated with proton pump inhibitors and IV fluids. On day 4 hemoglobin was in his baseline 14 g/dl and vitals were unremarkable. Pulmonology who then consulted IR for further intervention and biopsy of the lesion.

Upon pathology results, hematology/oncology was consulted and decided to begin treatment outpatient given hemodynamic stability at the moment and resolution of GI bleed after intervention. The patient was discharged after 7 days and was educated on the consequences of using NSAIDS and aspirin together. He was told to avoid these medications and was prescribed PPI for 6 weeks and follow up with his primary care physician. Patient was counseled on the importance of smoking cessation and goals of care were discussed with him and the family. They agreed to proceed with every treatment needed.

Challenge Questions

1. What paraneoplastic syndromes are associated with lung cancer?
   a. EPO, PTHrp, ACTH, Renin
   b. SIADH, Lamberton Eaton
   c. Renin, SIADH

2. Which of the following patients would benefit from lung cancer screening with an annual low-dose CT scan of the chest?
   a. Patient age 50-80 who has 20-pack-year history
   b. COPD patient on chronic O2 via nasal cannula
   c. Patient age 40-80 who has 15-pack-year history
   d. COPD patient with prior history of smoking 15 years ago.

3. Where are adenocarcinomas usually located in the lung?
   a. Centrally
   b. Peripherally
   c. Both, but usually peripheral

ABOUT THE AUTHOR

Dr. Luis Daniel Lugo, a Board-Certified Internist, specializes in Hospital Medicine. He received his medical degree from the renowned Saba University School of Medicine in the Netherlands. Following this, he undertook his Internal Medicine Residency at Roger Williams Medical Center, affiliated with the prestigious Boston University School of Medicine. Dr. Lugo further honed his expertise by completing a specialized fellowship program in Cardiovascular and Renal (CVR) at Bayer Pharmaceuticals, under the auspices of Rutgers University, Institute for Pharmaceutical Industry.

Beyond his medical qualifications, Dr. Lugo also holds a Master's degree in Business Administration with a specialization in Healthcare Management. His passion for education extends back to his early career as a high-school Chemistry teacher.

Before his tenure at Lakeland Regional Health, Dr. Lugo held the position of Associate Program Director for the Categorical Internal Medicine Residency Program at SUNY Downstate Medical Center, located in Brooklyn, New York. His dedication to service led him to work with veterans at the U.S. Department of Veterans Affairs in Brooklyn and with a diverse patient population at the Mount Sinai Health System in Manhattan.

In addition to his clinical work, Dr. Lugo's commitment to education has seen him serve as Clinical Associate Professor at both SUNY Downstate College of Medicine and Icahn School of Medicine at Mount Sinai, where he mentored numerous residents and students. His exceptional teaching skills have earned him multiple "Teacher of the Year" awards.